MY SUGAR FREE
BABY AND ME

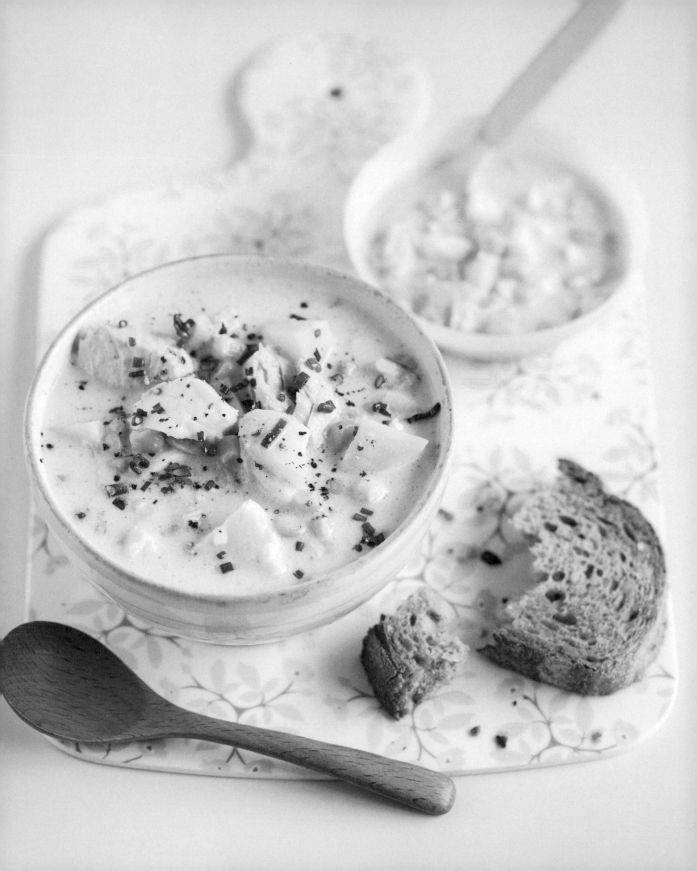

MY SUGAR FREE BABY AND ME

DR SARAH SCHENKER

BLOOMSBURY

LONDON · OXFORD · NEW YORK · NEW DELHI · SYDNEY

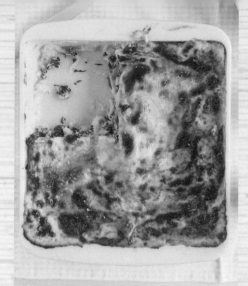

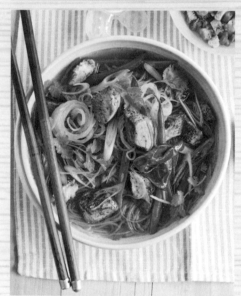

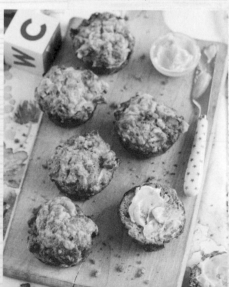

Bloomsbury Publishing, an imprint of Bloomsbury Publishing Plc

50 Bedford Square	1385 Broadway
London	New York
WC1B 3DP	NY 10018
UK	USA

www.bloomsbury.com

BLOOMSBURY and the Diana logo are trademarks of Bloomsbury Publishing Plc

First published 2017
© Dr Sarah Schenker, 2017

Photos ©
Adrian Lawrence Photography pp. 63, 66, 72, 77, 80, 85, 89, 93, 94, 98, 102, 107, 110, 113, 117,123, 126, 129, 134, 137, 143, 144, 149, 154, 159, 162, 165, 168, 173, 176, 177, 181, 184, 189, 192, 197 and 198 (c).
Getty Images pp. 15, 16, 26, 33, 36, 39, 42, 45, 47, 48, 50, 51, 52, 53, 54, 60, 65, 71, 86, 90, 101, 130, 132, 156, 161, 167, 171 and 182 (c).
Guy Baker pp. 7, 8, 11, 12, 25, 28, 31, 35, 40, 58, 104, 120 and 138.
Liz Dvorkin pp. 201

British Library Cataloguing-in-Publication Data
A catalogue record for this book is available from the British Library.

Library of Congress Cataloguing-in-Publication data has been applied for.

ISBN
Print: 978-1-4729-3900-5
ePDF: 978-1-4729-3902-9
ePub: 978-1-4729-3901-2

2 4 6 8 10 9 7 5 3 1

Design and illustration by Louise Turpin
Printed and bound in Great Britain by Bell & Bain Limited

Bloomsbury Publishing Plc makes every effort to ensure that the papers used in the manufacture of our books are natural, recyclable products made from wood grown in well-managed forests. Our manufacturing processes conform to the environmental regulations of the country of origin.

To find out more about our authors and books visit www.bloomsbury.com. Here you will find extracts, author interviews, details of forthcoming events and the option to sign up for our newsletters.

CONTENTS

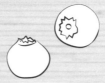

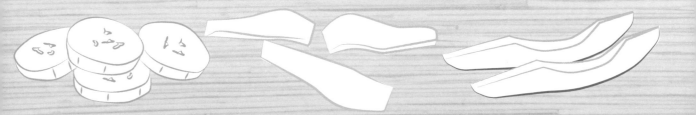

COOK'S NOTES

MEASUREMENTS

All spoon measures are rounded unless otherwise stated
- 1 tbsp is 15ml
- 1 tsp is 5ml

If you prefer to work in ounces:
- 1oz is 25g
- A pinch is approximately ¼ of a tsp
- A handful of herbs or leaves is approximately 25g

OVENS

All recipes were tested in a conventional oven. If using a fan-assisted oven, set the temperature 10 °C lower than stated in the recipes.

INGREDIENTS

- Use low salt stock cubes or gels.
- Use relatively fresh jars of spice, although they last for ages they lose a lot of their flavour the older they are.
- Use medium-sized eggs unless otherwise stated and when baking, remember to use room temperature eggs.
- Use grass fed cow's butter or you can substitute butter for coconut oil if you prefer.
- Use either olive or rapeseed oil unless otherwise stated. Rapeseed oil has a more delicate flavour.
- If using dried pulses (beans, chickpeas and lentils) soak overnight or for at least 8 hours.

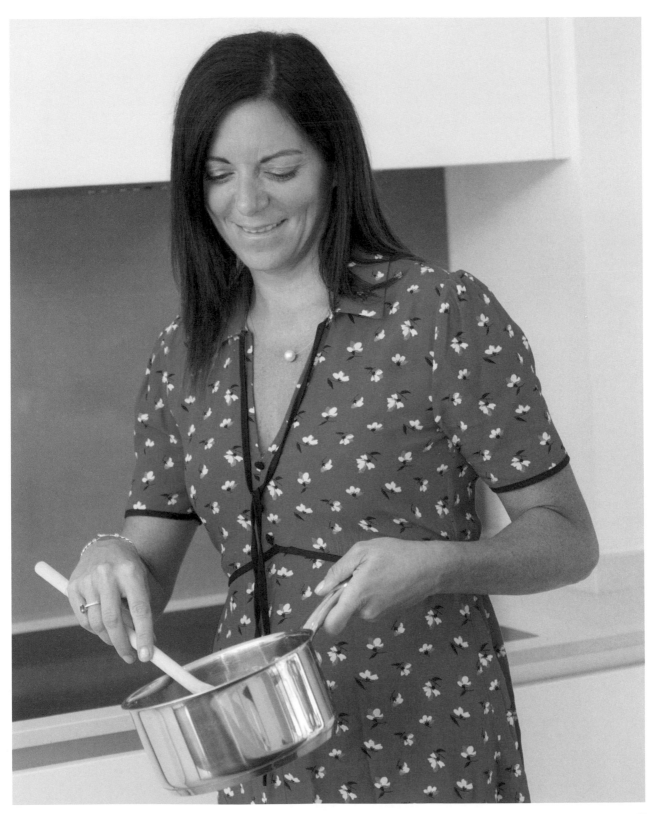

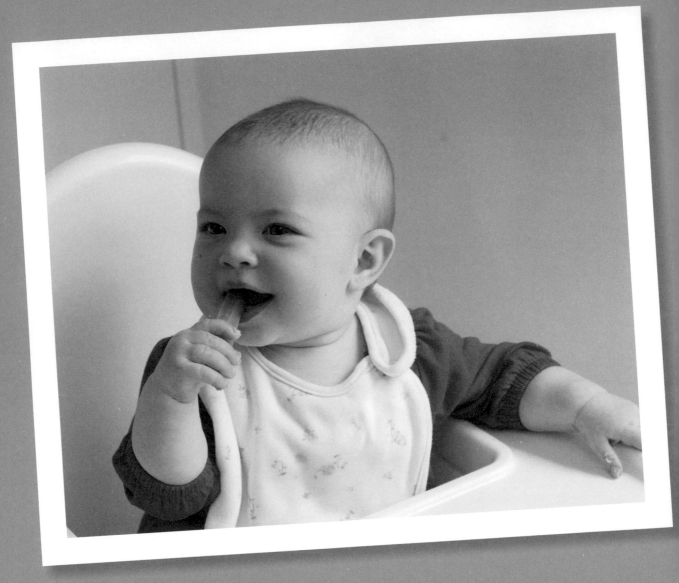

STARTING SOLIDS

Parents know that one of the best ways to give a baby a
great start in life is with wholesome homemade foods.
While ready made food is a convenience that any new
parent can appreciate, feeding everyday fresh foods is
the best way to teach a child healthy eating habits
and a love of good food from the very beginning.

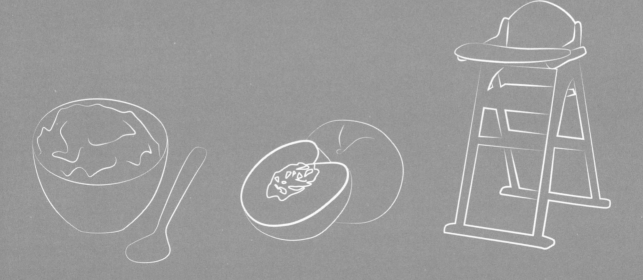

STARTING SOLIDS

As the mum of two lovely young boys I have been through the fun and antics of weaning twice, and as a dietitian I have helped and advised numerous new parents on weaning their babies. Many challenges can arise during this process and it is understandable to feel anxious or need some reassurance. This book is here to guide you through your weaning journey, making it fun, easy and above all healthy for both your baby and you.

Starting solids is one of the great milestones of your baby's first year of life. It is one of those subjects that everyone has an opinion about, along with the best wipes to use and whether your baby ought to be crawling by now.

One of the biggest questions is when to begin. Just a generation or two ago, babies were commonly started on solid foods at the tender age of 6 weeks, so don't be surprised if you hear that from a well-meaning grandma. The advice has changed, and experts now recommend exclusive breastfeeding (or formula feeding) for at least 17 weeks. This is because your baby's gut and the immune system are still somewhat under-developed at this stage. Some experts recommend that solids shouldn't be given until a baby is six months old, others say that it is acceptable to offer foods a little earlier, at four months, but warn that early introduction of foods has been linked to food intolerance, diabetes and obesity.

Parents often worry that their baby needs more to eat than just milk or formula before the age of six months, and a baby going through a growth spurt can certainly seem ravenous. But babies can usually thrive this long on a liquid diet alone. In fact, breast milk or formula should make up the majority of a baby's diet until his first birthday. Until then, rather than supplying your baby's primary source of nutrition, feeding solids is a way for parents to let their baby explore a world of new tastes, textures and temperatures; practise the skills of eating; and learn to enjoy and appreciate the social aspects of mealtimes.

No two babies are the same and ultimately you should follow your instincts about when to offer your baby his first taste of solid food. While I don't advocate starting on the very day he turns four months, I also don't think that waiting until the six-month mark is the right thing to do if all it does is cause misery and anxiety. Both of my boys started on solids aged around five to five-and-a-half months as they were showing clear signs that they were interested in food. If you are unsure your baby is ready, then leave it a little longer. A hungry

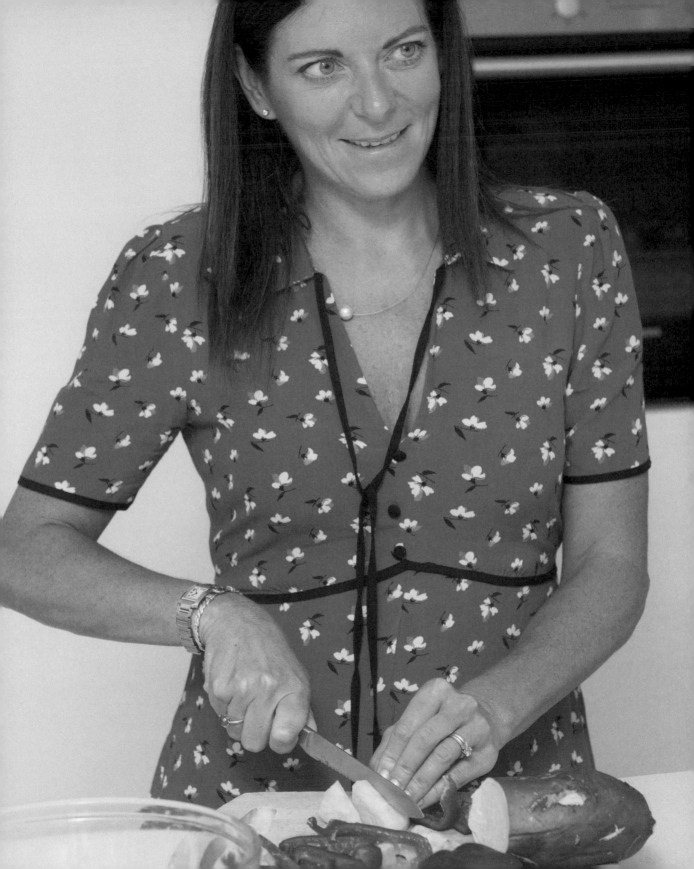

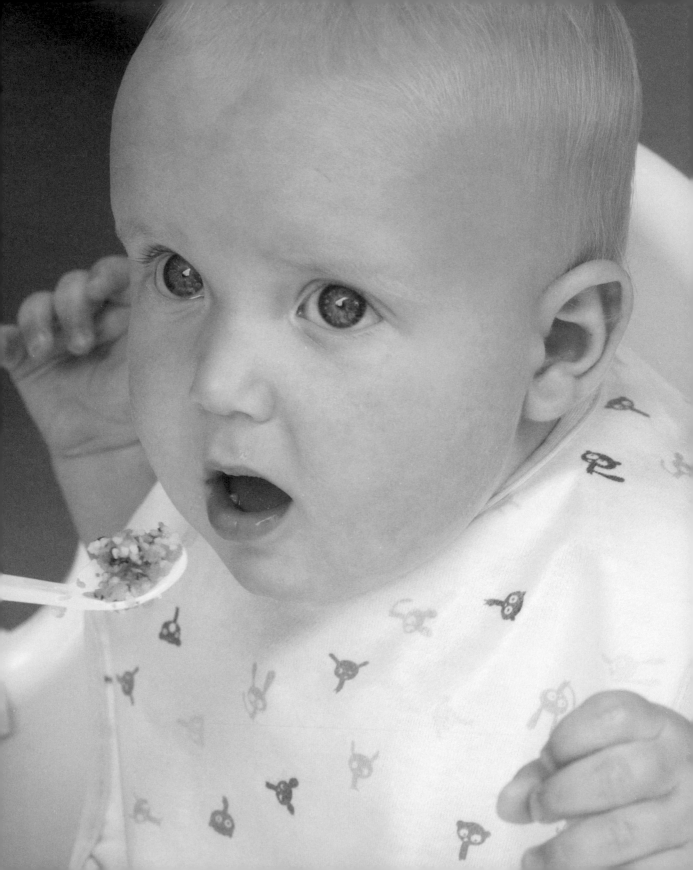

growing baby may just need additional feeds, and first solids are not designed to fill him up. You may very well find that the first time you offer baby a mouthful of mashed banana they turn away or spit it out (he may be more interested in playing with it), in which case you can leave it for a few days and try again.

FOLLOW BABY'S CUES

The best way to tell whether your baby is ready to start solids is to watch for cues. Here are some signs that show the time is right to begin offering food:

- Your baby is able to sit up well on her own without your assistance.
- Your baby is able to turn her head towards you when you are offering food (or turn it away).
- Your baby develops a persistent pattern of remaining hungry after the usual feeding.
- Your baby watches you when you eat and tries to grab your food.
- Your baby can swallow puréed food rather than reflexively spitting it out.

WHOLESOME AND HOME-MADE

New mums are sleep-deprived, dog-tired and even a little shell-shocked as they find their bundle of joy has turned their world upside down and is constantly demanding. On top of that your body is still recovering from the trauma of childbirth. However, finding the time to make wholesome meals for your baby and yourself should be a top priority. The foods you give your baby now, in the earliest months, will help shape your child's taste for many years to come. Moreover, choosing to eat the same good food will nourish and heal your body; give you sustained energy to get you through the day; provide nutrients to ensure a healthy supply of breast milk; and ensure good nutrition to balance hormones, which will impact on your ability to deal with tiredness, mood swings and the sensation of just feeling completely overwhelmed.

A friend of mine told me about the night her husband came home late from work to find her up to her elbows in fruit peelings as she made huge batches of purées, while polishing off a packet of Jaffa Cakes and a bottle of rosé! I also had a few moments when I thought I couldn't cope without wine and chocolate, but it tends to backfire, as the inevitable sore head the next day will be even harder to bear when you feel even more exhausted. Eating well now gives you more energy for your baby.

If you feed your baby only bland, processed baby food and cereals, your baby will become accustomed to bland, processed food. On the other hand, if you feed your baby a variety of fresh veg, fruit, grains, meat and fish flavoured with herbs and spices, you are priming his palate for a lifetime of healthy eating habits. And it's the same for you; if you rely on packets of biscuits and sugary drinks to get you through the day, all you are doing is creating a rollercoaster of energy highs and lows. Each time your energy levels crash, you'll reach for the next sugary snack and the whole process is repeated. This can have a disastrous result on your weight. I have often found with clients that the real damage to their weight happened after, not during pregnancy as they just didn't think about looking after themselves during such a hectic time.

If you are still breastfeeding, the body will draw on its supplies of nutrients to make good-quality nutritious breast milk for your baby, at your expense. Only in very extreme situations will the quality of the breast milk suffer. This is great for your baby but not for your body or your health. Not eating well will just exacerbate the tiredness, leave you feeling fatigued and run down, more vulnerable to colds and infections and probably quite emotional.

The odd pouch of ready-made baby food is not a terrible thing, I would certainly carry a few pouches in my changing bag if we were out and about, but the more food I made at home, the more I would double up so I could provide good food wherever we were. Once you've decided to start cooking, you may as well cook a batch of food and then it's so easy to make portable little meals, use clip-lock tubs and throw them into your bag.

The other issue with too much ready-made baby food is that you can fall into the trap of always buying the ones your baby likes the best and this does not help him develop a liking for a wide variety of flavours. Ready-made baby foods also lack variety of texture – even the ones that claim to be lumpy will always have exactly the same lumpiness and so do not get your baby used to different textures. Although you would be hard pushed to find any manufacturer who adds sugar, salt, additives or nasty fillers to their brand any more, making your own baby food will always be more nutritious. Some ready-made baby foods are heated to extremely high temperatures during processing, which destroys certain heat-sensitive vitamins to a much greater extent than home cooking does.

GO ORGANIC

To reduce your baby's exposure to toxins, choose organic ingredients when you can. If you find it is too expensive to buy everything organic, then just opt for organic on the thin-skinned fruit and veg such as apples, pears and potatoes, as these absorb pesticides more readily than thicker-skinned ones such as carrots and parsnips.

Chicken is likely to become a staple in your baby's diet as they get older. Aim to buy the best quality you can afford. Organic standards help to lower the risk of contamination and organic chicken tends to be nutritionally superior to non-organic chicken. Chickens that have experienced a high level of welfare contain more protein and fats that are better for the growth and development of your baby. Always choose eggs that have the Red Lion stamp.

 It is also a good idea to buy organic versions of fatty foods such as meats, dairy and oils, since pesticides and other environmental toxins tend to be stored in fat cells.

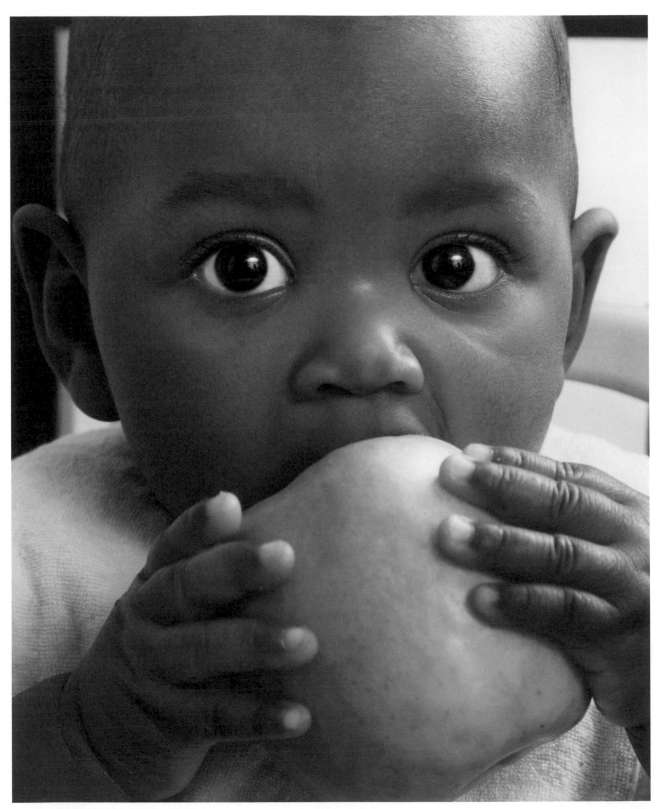

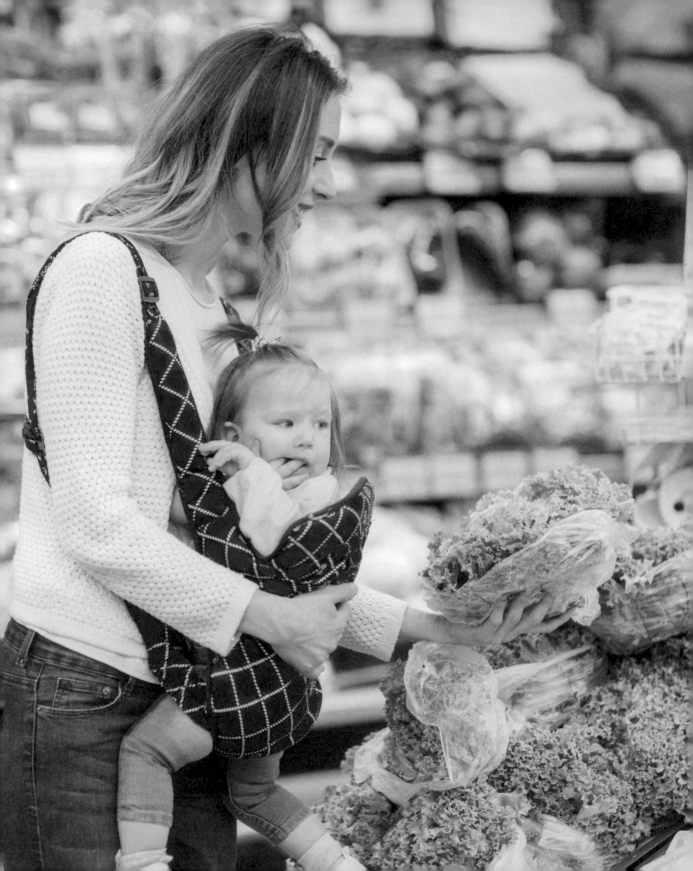

HOW TO BEGIN

At around six months your baby's digestive system is still developing, so the first foods you offer should be the ones that are most mild in flavour and easiest to digest. Introducing solids to your baby is a slow but enjoyable process of building a repertoire. With each new food you offer your baby, you are shaping her taste and testing her tolerance.

Some foods might not agree with her and may cause a tummy upset or even cause a rash, which is totally normal. This could be an immediate rash around the mouth or you may notice a small rash somewhere else on her body a few hours later. Don't be alarmed, this is a perfectly natural reaction to a first taste of a food. Just try a different food instead; you can offer the 'offending' food a bit later, when weaning is fully underway and you are unlikely to see the same reaction. New foods should be introduced one at a time as this gradual approach will make it easier to identify any 'culprit' foods.

Fruit allergy is quite rare in babies, but there are a handful of fruits that can cause a mild reaction by irritating the skin around the mouth. These include kiwi fruit, strawberries, raspberries and oranges. This is nothing to worry about and the rash should calm down quite quickly. Simply avoid this fruit for a while. You may be able to introduce it once your baby is eating a full range of foods or it may continue to cause a problem until your child is older.

Some babies will have delayed allergic reactions to foods and these are much harder to spot as the symptoms tend to last longer and be more persistent than immediate reactions. They may include reflux, colic, diarrhoea, constipation and eczema. Some of these symptoms can be caused by conditions other than allergies, so it is important to see your GP for a diagnosis.

WHAT TO DO IF YOUR BABY HAS A SERIOUS ALLERGIC REACTION

If your baby experiences an immediate allergic reaction the first symptoms you are likely to see include watering and itchy eyes and nose, itchy mouth, a skin rash or hives, swollen lips and eyes, possibly followed by vomiting and diarrhoea. More severe reactions are much rarer and involve wheezing, breathing difficulties, throat and tongue swelling and a drop in blood pressure. This is known as anaphylaxis and can be life threatening so call an ambulance immediately.

FIRST TASTES

These foods are great as first tastes as they are easily digestible and nutritious and usually agree with your baby:

- Sweet potato
- Butternut squash
- Potato
- Cooked apple

- Cooked pear
- Banana
- Avocado
- Rice

- Millet
- Barley

If your baby suffers from colic, these foods might make the problem worse since they produce more gas, so are less suitable as first tastes:

- Peas
- Beans
- Lentils

- Broccoli
- Cabbage
- Cauliflower

- Cucumber
- Onion

There will be plenty of opportunities to introduce these foods once weaning is underway.
   Most new mums will buy a highchair and there are many styles and types to choose from, easy clean plastic, wooden step types that pull up to the table or large comfy padded ones

ADDITIONAL EQUIPMENT FOR WEANING

While you should certainly expect some mess during weaning, think spaghetti on the walls and peas on the floor, you can make things a little easier for yourself by having the right weaning equipment to hand. You'll probably have most of what you need in the house, but there are a few extra things that are worth buying as they will come in handy:

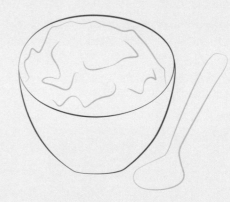

- A few strong brightly coloured plastic spoons (the bright colours will catch your baby's attention) small enough for a little mouth

- A colourful plastic bowl – preferably with a sucker on the bottom to prevent upsets

- Plenty of bibs and clean cloths

- A floor mat to stand a highchair on

- A food blender/processor

- Bendy ice-trays for storing extra portions

- Clip-lock tubs to store extra food

that can fold away. However, you may like to consider a seat that attaches to the table or that straps onto one of your usual kitchen/dining room chairs instead of a freestanding highchair. This allows your baby to feel part of the eating experience because they are eating from the same table as you.

Hook-on chairs are useful when space is limited and tend to cost less than standard highchairs. They are also portable so they're useful for eating out. However not all hook-on chairs work on every table, so you need to check before you buy.

CUPS

If you have been bottle feeding, it's a good idea to introduce a trainer cup from about six months. By the time your baby is one, they should have stopped using bottles with teats. This prevents your baby developing a habit of comfort sucking. It is reported that comfort sucking is the biggest cause of tooth decay in young children.

Choose a trainer cup that is open, maybe with a spout, and not a lidded cup with a teat as this will help your baby to learn to sip rather than suck, which is better for their teeth. When using a trainer cup, don't put anything in it other than formula milk, breast milk or water.

A QUESTION OF SWEETNESS

We are born with a sweet tooth (even before we start teething!). It is part of our ancient genetic make-up that enables us to survive. Sweetness was a sign that a food was ripe and safe to eat and would be a good source of energy when food was scarce. Breastmilk has the perfect sweetness and formula milk is designed to be the same, enticing your baby to start feeding straight after birth and getting on with the business of surviving! So it is natural that your baby is more likely to be tempted with a spoonful of mashed banana or puréed apple as a first taste than with puréed cauliflower. However, it is important not to let the sweetness of your baby's food intensify. If everything you offer is fruity and sweet, your baby's liking for sweetness will build, so it is sensible to introduce some less sweet foods such as potato and avocado in the early stages.

Another reason for not overdoing the fruit is the concern that we could overload the baby's system with too much fruit sugar. The natural sugar in milk is lactose, and once weaning starts this is often replaced by fructose as a source of energy. Studies in animals have looked at the impact of high doses of fructose being introduced during weaning and found potentially harmful effects on the liver and insulin sensitivity. Eating too much fructose has been linked with rising levels of obesity and type 2 diabetes. This doesn't mean you should not offer fruit, quite the opposite – fruits are a valuable source of nutrients for your baby – it's just a question of striking the right balance.

FOODS TO AVOID

There are certain foods that you should not give to your baby before he is six months and other foods that he can't have before his first birthday.

FOOD	SAFE BEFORE 6 MONTHS?	SAFE AT 6 MONTHS?	SAFE BEFORE 12 MONTHS?	SAFE AT 12 MONTHS?
Cow's milk, yogurt, cheese	✘	✔ For small amounts used in cooking	✔ But cow's milk should not be given as a main drink	✔ Can be given as a drink
Goat's milk and soya, nut and other alternative 'milks'	✘	✔ For small amounts in cooking	✔ But not as a main drink	✔
Brie, Camembert and other mould-ripened cheeses	✘ Because these cheeses pose a greater risk of food poisoning	✘	✘	✔
Eggs	✘	✔ If well cooked	✔ If you want to give soft-boiled eggs, look for those with a Red Lion stamp or equivalent mark denoting that the eggs have been produced to the highest standard and are from hens that have been vaccinated against salmonella	
Bread, pasta and wheat products	✘	✔ But not as a very first food, better from 7 months	✔	✔

FOODS TO AVOID continued

FOOD	SAFE BEFORE 6 MONTHS?	SAFE AT 6 MONTHS?	SAFE BEFORE 12 MONTHS?	SAFE AT 12 MONTHS?
Prawns and other shellfish	✘	✔ But not as a very first food, better from 7 months	✔ But observe especially good food hygiene because these foods pose a particular risk of food poisoning	✔ But observe especially good food hygiene
Marlin, swordfish, shark	✘	✘ These fish contain high levels of mercury and should be avoided by babies and young children	✘	✘
Salmon and other fish	✘	✔ These fish are an excellent source of omega-3 fatty acids	✔	✔
Smoked salmon and other smoked fish	✘	✘ Because they are high in salt	✘	✔
Peanut butter and other nut butters	✘	✔	✔	✔
Whole nuts	✘	✘ Whole nuts pose a significant choking hazard	✘	✘
Sesame seeds	✘	✔	✔	✔

FOODS TO AVOID continued

FOOD	SAFE BEFORE 6 MONTHS?	SAFE AT 6 MONTHS?	SAFE BEFORE 12 MONTHS?	SAFE AT 12 MONTHS?
Honey	✗	✗ Because there is a small risk of Cholstridium botulism	✗	✔
Salt	✗	✗ Baby's kidneys are under developed	✗	✗
Citrus fruit	✗	✔	✔	✔
Kiwi	✗	✗ Not as a first food, because small risk of fruit allergy	✔ From 9 months	✔
Strawberries	✗	✗ Not as a first food, because small risk of food allergy	✔ From 9 months	✔
Tea	✗	✗ Because it contains caffeine, which disrupts your baby's sleep, and tannins that make it harder for your baby to absorb iron from food	✗	✗
Coffee	✗	✗ Because it contains caffeine, which disrupts your baby's sleep, and tannins that make it harder for your baby to absorb iron from food	✗	✗

INTRODUCING NUTS

I am a big fan of nuts of all varieties because they are one of the most nutritious foods available to us. They provide protein, healthy fats and an array of vitamins and minerals. Naturally you can't offer your baby whole nuts as there is a serious risk that they could choke, however, nut butters, including peanut butter can and should be offered. Nut butters are energy dense, meaning a little goes a long way and this is important for small tummies that need regular filling but not over filling. Choose brands that do not have salt or sugar added, or try making your own by simply roasting on a baking tray for a few minutes and blitzing in a food processor. Blitz well until smooth, so there are no hidden big chunks and add a drop of oil to make a smoother consistency.

If you ate peanuts during your pregnancy it won't affect your baby's chance of developing a peanut allergy. However, if you have a family history of peanut allergy or other food allergies, or your baby has already developed an allergy such as eczema or a food allergy, it is best not to introduce peanuts at this stage, and seek advice from your health visitor or GP.

CONSISTENCY

The first meals you give your baby should have a very runny consistency – in other words more liquid than solid. Babies have a protective reflex, which means the tongue will thrust to keep food (and non-food items) out of their mouths before they are able to manage them without choking. This will prevent them from swallowing thick solids. Swallowing food is a skill your baby needs to develop bit by bit. Use a food processor or hand-held blender to purée a food such as cooked apple and then add a little of your breast or formula milk to make it more runny.

HOW OFTEN AND HOW MUCH

Keep in mind that *for the first year*, breast milk or formula should continue to be your baby's primary source of nutrition, although from six months your baby starts to need iron from food, as breast milk alone won't give him enough. Offer a feeding of breast milk or formula before offering food, so that the food does not replace the milk but merely supplements it. A good idea is to offer some food midway through a milk feed so that your baby is not too full up to be interested in what is being offered. To begin with just offer food once a day: the middle of the day is a good time, when your baby is at her most alert and energetic. Let your baby decide whether or how much he eats. This could be anything from a couple of spoonfuls to a small bowl. Just like adults, your baby's appetite will vary from day to day. Losing interest, turning the head away, pushing the spoon away or spitting out food are all signs that your baby has had enough. It doesn't matter whether or not your baby has finished all the food in his bowl, you can just try again with a fresh batch later or the next day.

THE NEXT STEPS

At first your baby's puréed food should remain quite runny, but each week you can gradually make it thicker. Offer your baby different consistencies by mixing smooth purées with chunkier mashes, such as pear purée with mashed potato or apple purée with butternut squash mash. Or you can thicken a thin purée with baby rice and other baby cereals. At around seven to eight months your baby will start to pick up and chew soft finger foods, which he can mash well with his gums even before he has many teeth.

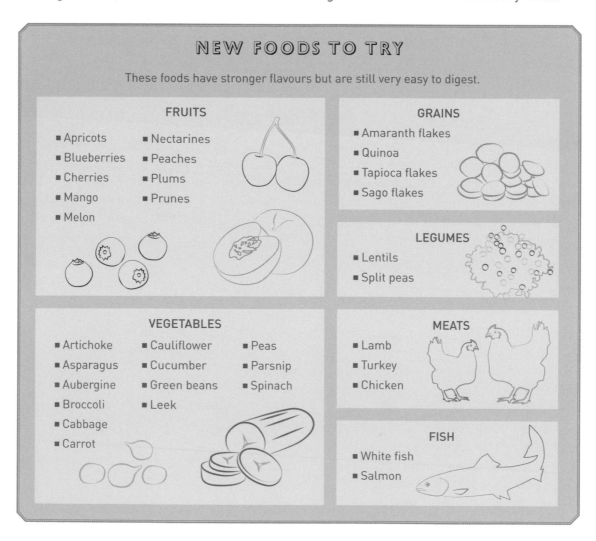

NEW FOODS TO TRY

These foods have stronger flavours but are still very easy to digest.

FRUITS

- Apricots
- Blueberries
- Cherries
- Mango
- Melon
- Nectarines
- Peaches
- Plums
- Prunes

GRAINS

- Amaranth flakes
- Quinoa
- Tapioca flakes
- Sago flakes

LEGUMES

- Lentils
- Split peas

VEGETABLES

- Artichoke
- Asparagus
- Aubergine
- Broccoli
- Cabbage
- Carrot
- Cauliflower
- Cucumber
- Green beans
- Leek
- Peas
- Parsnip
- Spinach

MEATS

- Lamb
- Turkey
- Chicken

FISH

- White fish
- Salmon

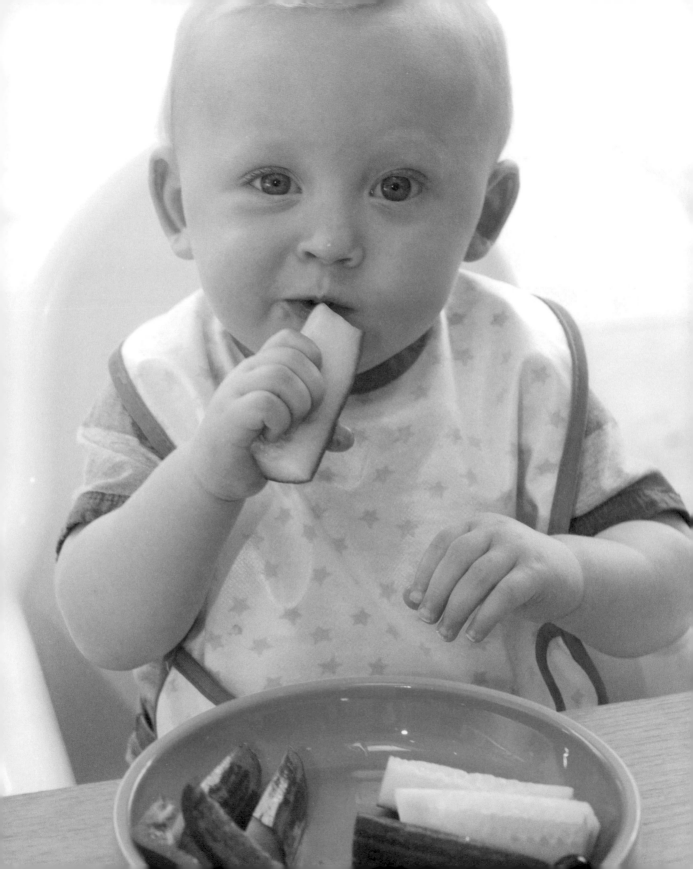

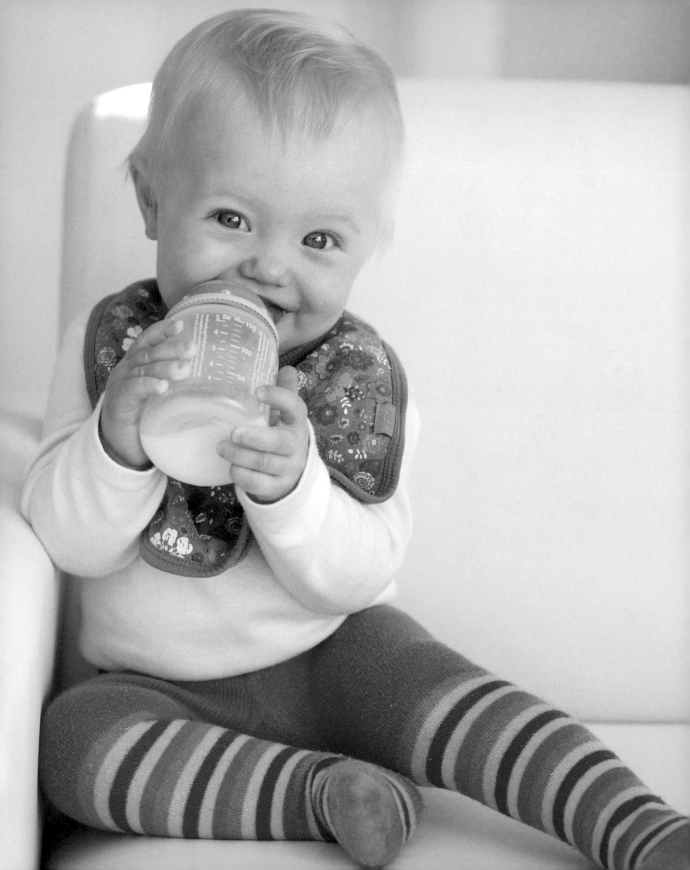

From six months, start offering your baby an additional daily meal each month, so that by eight months she is eating three times a day. Be guided by your baby's appetite and allow your baby to eat as much of her solid food as she likes, ideally a short while after she has finished a milk feed. This means that the breast or formula milk remains the main source of nutrition for your baby and she will not be over-hungry or tetchy when you offer her a meal.

Continue to introduce new foods and start mixing them together with other foods your baby has already tried. There are bound to be a couple of foods that your baby won't like the look, smell or flavour of. Don't force him to eat it, just try again another day, maybe mixed with a different food. It's common for babies to accept a food only after it becomes familiar, and it may take as many as 10–15 tries before this happens!

WHAT TO DO IF YOUR BABY IS CHOKING

The NHS Choices website gives the following advice:

- If you can see the object, try to remove it. Don't poke blindly or repeatedly with your fingers. You could make things worse by pushing the object further in and making it harder to remove.

- If your baby is coughing allow them to continue and don't leave them.

- If your baby becomes silent and can't breathe in properly get help immediately.

- If your child is still conscious, but not coughing, try giving them back blows.

- Sit down and lay your baby face down along your thighs, supporting their head with your hand.

- Give up to five sharp back blows with the heel of one hand in the middle of the back between the shoulder blades.

- If back blows don't relieve the choking and your baby is still conscious, try giving

abdominal thrusts. This will create an artificial cough, increasing pressure in the chest and helping to dislodge the object.

- Lay your baby face up along the length of your thighs.

- Find the breastbone, and place two fingers in the middle.

- Give five sharp chest thrusts (pushes), compressing the chest by about a third.

- Following chest or abdominal thrusts, reassess your child to see if the object has been dislodged.

- If not, continue this routine until help comes and don't leave your child.

- If your baby becomes unconscious with choking put them on a firm, flat surface and dial 999.

- Don't leave your child at any stage.

BECOMING A FOOD EXPLORER

As your baby starts to enjoy his meals, he will become an ever-more active participant, trying to grab the spoon to feed himself, dropping food on the floor, throwing it at you and spreading it in his hair. Believe it or not these are all encouraging signs that your baby is well on the way to becoming self-sufficient at the table, so rather than worry about the mess, embrace it (or at least try to...)!

Let your baby take the spoon, or give her a second spoon to play with while you feed her. Allow plenty of time as at this stage mealtimes will be more chaotic. Have your meals at the same time and swap spoonfuls of foods so your baby experiences the pleasure of sharing and enjoying food together.

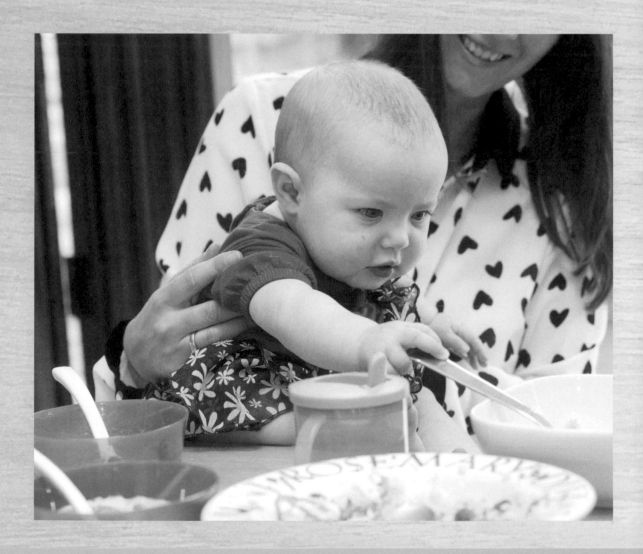

Don't worry too much about offering perfectly balanced meals at this stage. Instead, use this time to introduce as many different tastes, textures and flavours as you can. A reminder – until the age of 1 year, your baby's main source of nutrition is his milk feed which is providing the vitamins, minerals, fats and protein your baby needs to grow and develop.

When three meals a day plus milk feeds no longer seems to satisfy his appetite you can start to introduce snacks. These could be leftovers from a previous meal or sugar-free finger foods. Always try to make time to stop what you are doing, move to the table or another part of the room away from any distractions, such as the television or toys, and focus on the food. This will prevent your baby becoming a mindless eater. Offer a small cup of water with the snack.

STRONGER-TASTING FOODS TO TRY

There is no nutritional reason why you can't offer these foods from seven months, but their flavours may be too strong for your baby. Gauge their reaction and go at their pace.

- Beetroot
- Celery
- Garlic
- Onions
- Peppers
- Spring onions
- Berries
- Coconut
- Grapefruit
- Kiwi
- Oranges
- Papaya
- Pineapple

Your baby's tastes may start to change and no doubt she will be exercising her own will, so don't be surprised if she rejects a food that she used to enjoy. Try offering the rejected food in a new form, such as spread on bread or mixed with different foods, and don't react – instead keep a cheerful expression. She may well change her mind again tomorrow or next week, but if she gets a disapproving reaction from you (and your baby will be an expert at reading your reactions by now) it will only encourage her to carry on refusing.

Offer thicker and chunkier textures by coarsely mashing or chopping food rather than blending it. A combination of the two can also work quite well, for instance blend some chicken and spinach and combine with some roughly mashed sweet potato.

USING HERBS AND SPICES

Processed baby foods can be very bland, but your baby's home-made food doesn't have to be the same. Babies in many cultures are introduced to strong herbs and spices early on, so don't be afraid to try strong flavours. Be guided by your own diet, culture and your baby. Treat herbs and spices like any other ingredient, introducing them one at a time, starting with milder ones such as dill and cinnamon and moving on to the more pungent ones as her palate develops.

FAST TRACK WEANING

Although it may seem there is a lot of information on weaning to absorb, try not to feel overwhelmed or anxious about it. As a new parent your instincts are strong: trust them and remember there is no perfect process. All babies are different and it is highly unlikely you could cause any harm by acting intuitively.

I remember when my son had just started weaning and I was having a mummy-and-baby lunch with my new friends. There I was trying to spoon mushy avocado into his mouth when he suddenly grabbed a big chunk of French baguette from my plate. Everyone was looking at me to see what I would do, but I felt Daniel had made a clear statement – he wanted my bread! We are lucky enough not to suffer from any food allergies in our family, so I decided to let him enjoy it. He happily gummed and sucked on it in between mouthfuls of the avocado.

It is this half-and-half approach I favour, as opposed to completely spoon-fed or exclusive baby-led weaning. It's a sort of fast-track weaning, which means your baby doesn't get bored on weeks and weeks of nothing but purées, but equally your baby receives adequate amounts of nutrients from their food, which is difficult to achieve with exclusive baby-led weaning.

Once your baby can safely swallow and does not gag on soft, runny food, you can give him small pieces of food to hold in his hand as you feed him. He is more likely to squish them, smear them or rub them in his or your hair than actually eat them, but he will love holding them and trying to feed himself. Give him slices of soft pear or avocado, small pieces of soft banana or skinless strips of cucumber to try. Also give him a spoon to hold. He won't have the skills to feed himself, but he will love having a go and making a mess.

Your new role as a mum can be a real leveller, especially if you have achieved and succeeded in your career. The perception that you have somehow 'failed' to feed or control your baby, added to the broken sleep, changed body and all the new stuff in your life can be quite overwhelming, but feeding your baby is neither a competition or a project to deliver. It's a special time to enjoy together and build a lasting bond. You're Mum and you know your baby better than anyone else, so as much as you can go with the flow and trust your instincts.

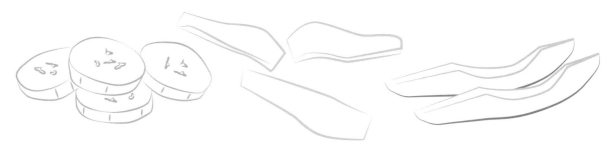

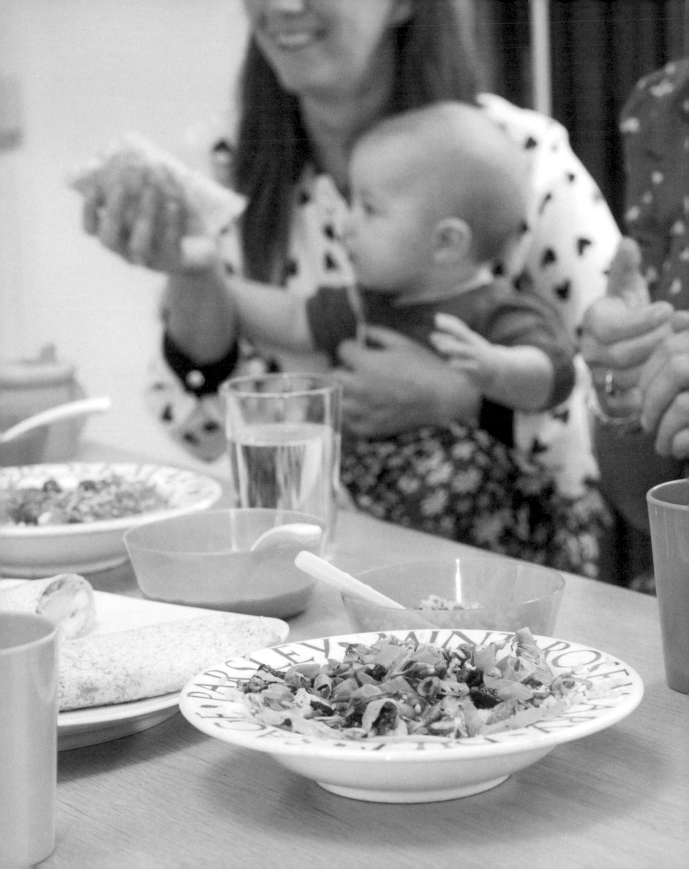

FINGER FOODS & CHUNKIER TEXTURES

At around nine months babies start to develop their pincer grip – using their thumb and finger to pick things up. This is an important new skill for your baby to develop and food is the perfect thing to practise with. At meal times, spread some items on the table (or high-chair tray) for your baby to pick up. Good things to try include:

- Cooked veg sticks
- Chunks of avocado
- Slices of soft fruit, such as pear, banana or melon
- Fingers of buttered toast or bread
- Berries and halved grapes*
- Cooked pasta shapes
- Chopped hard-boiled egg
- Sugar-free cereal shapes
- Real meals

> * Whole grapes pose a particular choking hazard, since they are the perfect size and shape to completely block the airway. Current advice is to slice grapes in half for children up to the age of five.

As your baby approaches his first birthday, he will be eating a wide variety of foods with coarser textures and he'll be more interested than ever in what you are eating, taking food from your plate and feeding his food to you. This behaviour is his natural instinct to bond with you and the rest of the family through food, so don't miss this opportunity to enjoy food together.

Your baby may be starting to develop a strong liking for her favourite foods and refuse others that she previously liked. A good strategy now is to offer familiar foods alongside new ones and to place dishes in the middle of the table and let other members of the family help themselves. Watching you or an older brother or sister tucking into a new dish will almost certainly have the effect of making your baby want it.

The more flavours your baby experiences early on, the more likely he is to come back to eating a wide range of foods later, even if he goes through the inevitable fussy stage.

Your baby is much more active now and will be constantly on the go, climbing, exploring and never in one place for long. This means her energy demands have shot up and she will need a constant supply of energy to support this. She will need three meals a day, plus healthy snacks between meals and her usual three or four milk feeds, but don't despair if she takes less milk now.

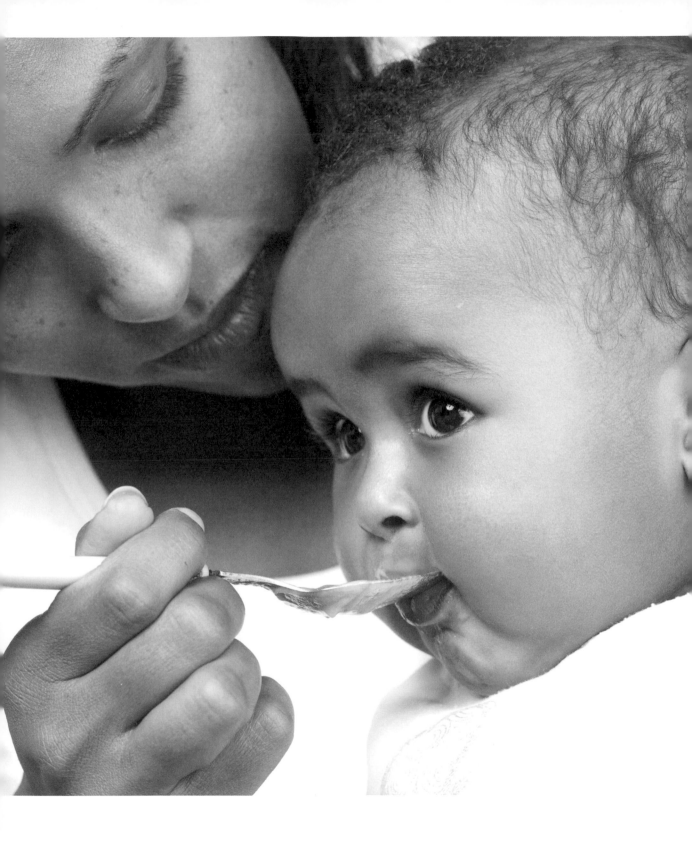

PORTABLE SNACKS

Offering a variety of snacks to your baby is important for two reasons: firstly it helps her to strengthen her fine motor skills and develop her pincer grip; secondly, it encourages her to try a wide range of different tastes and textures. I'm a firm believer that giving your baby a snack should be an eating event in that where possible you both stop what you are doing and focus on enjoying the snack, this is crucial in preventing the habit of mindless eating. It's ideal if you can sit down together at the table and turn off all distractions. However, the reality is you do need some healthy portable snacks to offer when you are out and about. Wherever you might be and whatever you are doing, try not to get into the habit of opening a packet of 'baby snacks' and just handing them mindlessly one at a time. They are usually nothing more than brightly coloured puffed cereals which have scant nutritional benefit other than to act as a filler. Chopped fruit and veg is one of the best options, it takes a bit more effort as you have to prepare it before you leave and it doesn't always travel well in bags, so it is worth investing in a few clip-lock tubs.

A few ideas:
- Slices of melon, avocado, peach, mango and pear
- Pieces of cooked veg (leftover from the night before) such as sticks of carrot, diced new potatoes, slices of sweet potato and spears of asparagus
- Fingers of soft wholegrain bread spread with soft cheese
- Soft scotch pancakes spread with smooth peanut butter
- Fingers of malt loaf spread with butter or soft cheese (NB: malt loaf does contain a little sugar, but the content is very low)
- Mini falafels
- Sliced omelette (it takes only minutes to whip up an omelette at home, slice it up and it's a great snack for later)
- Cubes of mild cheese.

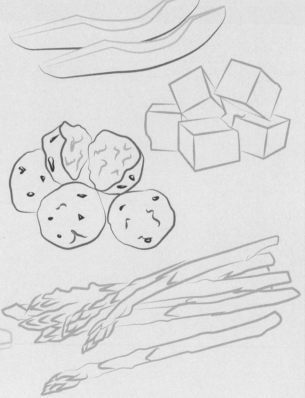

NUTRITIONAL NEEDS

From the time weaning starts your baby will receive 100 per cent of their nutritional needs from their milk and the aim is that by the time they have passed their first birthday and are approaching their second, they will receive most of their nutritional needs from a balanced diet (which will still include milk – either their usual milk or as cow's milk). It's a gradual transition from one to the other and somewhere in the middle there is a 50:50 split between their usual milk and solid foods providing the nutrition.

The average six-month-old baby requires about 550–600 calories a day, at one year the average requirement is around 700–750, and at two years 1000–1200 calories a day. These are average figures and you don't need to dwell on them or see them as targets, just allow

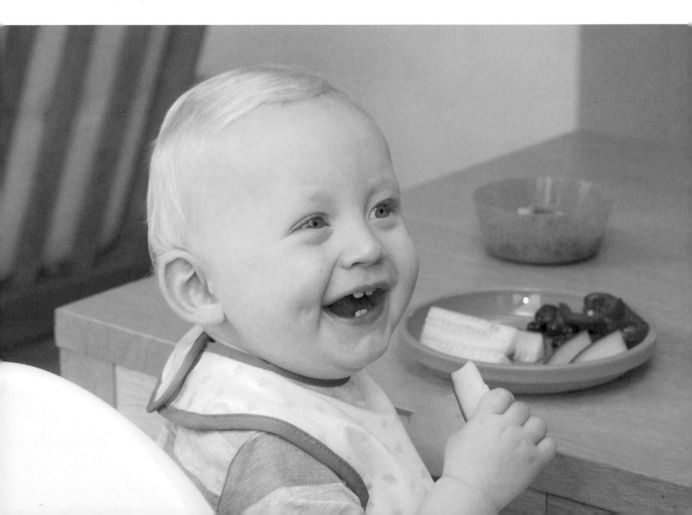

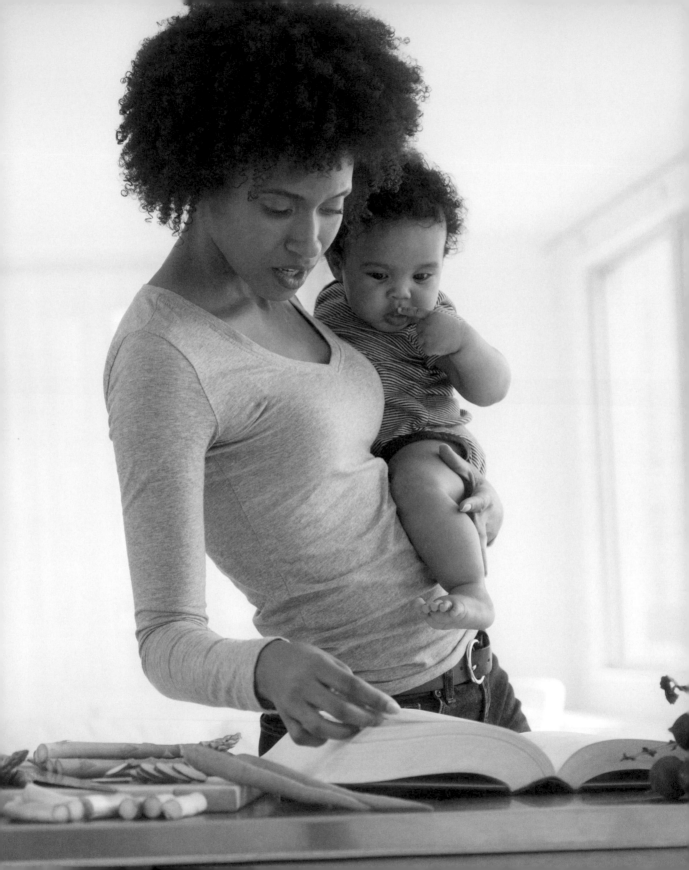

your baby's appetite to be the guide. Some days they will eat more than others and sometimes, just like anyone else, they will eat less. So long as your baby is growing and putting on weight in line with the trajectory on the growth charts, you can be confident they are getting enough and meeting their nutritional needs.

TEMPTING A FUSSY EATER

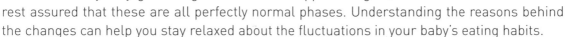

There will be times when you despair as your baby may go through a fussy stage, rejecting previously firm favourites as they learn to exercise their free will and show you who is boss! They may become fascinated with a certain food and only want to eat that one or they may go through a lull in their appetite. Again, rest assured that these are all perfectly normal phases. Understanding the reasons behind the changes can help you stay relaxed about the fluctuations in your baby's eating habits.

It's natural for a baby to reject bitter flavours: it's an ancient self-protective instinct. Blend stronger-flavoured vegetables with softer, sweeter flavours such as spinach with blueberries. Your baby's taste buds are sharper and more numerous than your own, so food will taste much more intense to them.

It's also helpful to remember that your baby does not grow at an even rate – they will go through growth spurts and growth lulls and their appetite will reflect this. They may seem ravenous for a couple of days and then a few days or a week later seem disinterested in anything you offer.

Your baby can become easily overwhelmed by change, so try not to offer too many new foods with different smells, colours and textures too quickly. Also pick your moments wisely when it comes to introducing something new. Your baby is more likely to try it if they are alert and happy rather than tired and grizzly.

Aim to strike a happy balance between routine and progression. Routine is important to babies as it makes them feel safe and secure, but rigid routine inhibits progress and weaning is a progress. Plan your day but allow some flexibility with the timings of feeding, or you will just build a rod for your back and may find that your routine stops you enjoying trips to the park, outings with other mums or baby yoga classes. I've heard stories of mums so fixated by routine they have attempted to feed their baby in the dark at baby cinema!

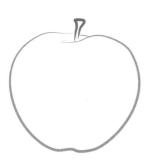

As frustrated as you might feel, try to avoid mealtime battles and never use food as reward or punishment. Avoid this bad habit from the beginning and you won't use it as your child becomes older. The best tactic is to keep the mood upbeat and let your baby see you eating and enjoying the same good foods.

SPOON-FED VS BABY-LED WEANING

There are many schools of thought when it comes to weaning, but the two most obvious camps are spoon-feeding vs baby-led weaning, both of which have their advantages. Puréed or well-mashed food is an obvious bridge between liquid and solid foods. It's also easy for you to see how much your baby is eating if you spoon-feed him, and you have greater control over what and how much (without force-feeding) your baby has at every meal. By six months, babies can take food off a spoon using their upper lip, rather than sucking the food off. By eight months, babies can chew and swallow foods with lumps, so it makes sense to adjust the consistency of their food as they develop. Baby-led weaning (BLW), on the other hand, means forgetting purées and weaning spoons, and simply letting your baby feed himself.

Many parents follow BLW without even thinking about it. This is particularly the case with second or later children. Babies love to copy their older siblings – they often try to grab food from other children's plates, happy to feed themselves just like their big brother or sister does. With BLW you need to be able to offer your baby a selection of nutritious finger foods suitable for his age. The easiest finger foods for babies are those that are cut into batons, or have a natural handle, such as cooked broccoli spears. This is because when your baby first tries solids, he won't yet have developed a pincer grip. The pincer grip enables him to pick up food between his thumb and forefinger. He will start to develop this skill over the next few months, but to begin with he can only clasp foods in his fists. He may grab pieces of food with his fist and start to suck on them, but you might find he is more likely just to play with them.

BLW gives babies the chance to explore foods for themselves, which means they can cope with different food textures from the beginning of weaning. Parents who have tried BLW are generally passionate about its benefits. They say their babies will eat anything and everything, which helps to take the worry out of starting solids. But although there's plenty of anecdotal evidence about BLW, not much formal research has been done.

One study did find that babies who are allowed to feed themselves from the beginning of weaning are more likely to join in with family mealtimes and eat a wide range of family foods early on. Another study found that BLW encourages babies to choose healthier foods, which could protect against obesity in childhood.

However, there are disadvantages, the most important of which is that BLW is unlikely to provide good nutrition as the process is very messy, and there is a lot of waste. If most of your baby's food ends up on the floor, there will be a limit to the number of nutrients he can get from his food.

Babies may find it hard to chew on some finger foods, such as well-cooked meat, which is a good source of iron – something that your baby needs to obtain from food from the age of six months. A spoon-fed baby would receive this in the form of palatable puréed meat, but a BLW baby runs the risk of missing out on this valuable source of iron.

The official advice is to give your baby well-mashed or puréed foods at the beginning of weaning, as well as finger food. The Department of Health, the European Union, and the World Health Organisation all recommend this.

I personally think it's important to give your baby a variety of textures, which includes sloppy foods as well as finger foods, so they receive the correct nutrition but also experience a wide range of textures and tastes.

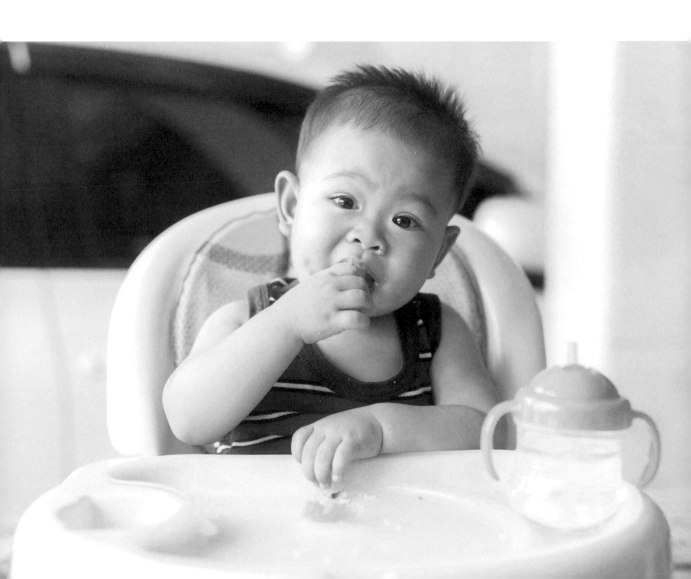

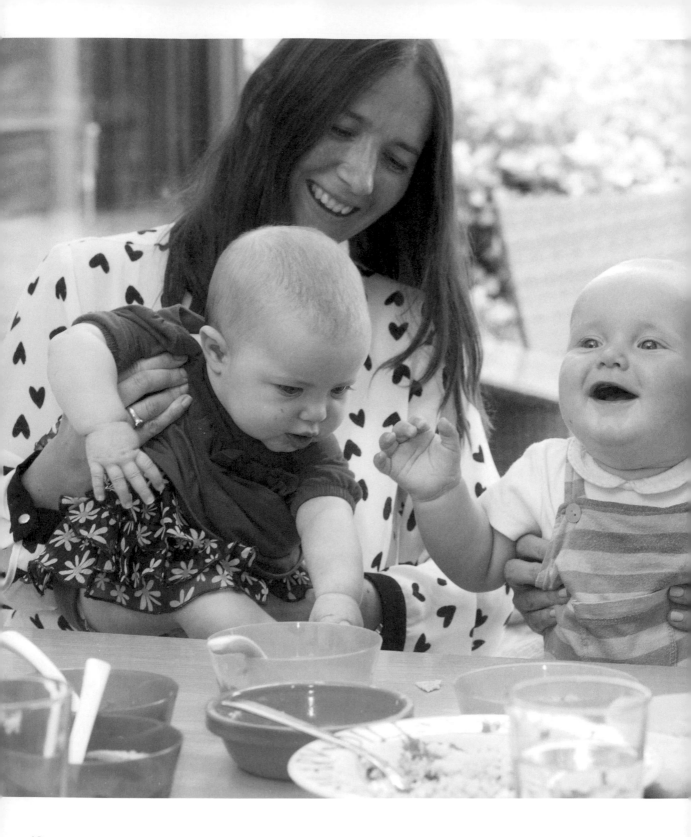

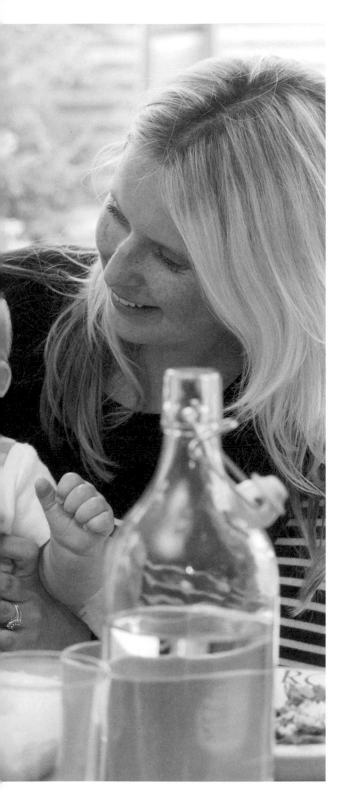

WHY YOU SHOULD EAT TOGETHER

Eating together and sharing food is one of life's real pleasures and so this should start from weaning.

A baby's first experience of food is so important to help develop adventurous tastes and avoid fussiness, so it needs to be social and inclusive. If they're eating alongside others, your baby will naturally copy other people, and eat a broader range of foods and develop better eating habits. Many babies sit in their highchairs with nobody else eating, while they are spoon-fed and wiped by an anxious mother, who might be worrying about mess or how much their little one is eating. Put yourself in their shoes for a minute. Such a stressful environment does not make for a lovely first-time experience of food and eating.

In addition, there are huge benefits for you if you eat with your baby. You are lovingly preparing wholesome healthy foods, which will do you just as much good as your baby. The better you eat, the better you will feel. This will help you deal with the tiredness, improve your mood and give you the energy you need to take on the challenges of the day.

LOOKING AFTER YOU

Eating with, and the same foods, as your baby will give you the opportunity to nourish your body. Your body has been on an incredible journey as it changed through pregnancy, experienced the trauma of childbirth and six months on is still recovering. What you eat can make a real difference to the healing process.

The foods you offer your baby are packed full of important vitamins and minerals he needs to grow and stay healthy and you need the same. These foods will help to reduce inflammation (caused by stress and trauma) and give your body nutrients so that it can heal and replenish lost energy. Eating a variety of foods will also help provide your body with a wide range of natural substances often termed phytochemicals. This includes substances such as flavanoids and anthocyanins, which have health-boosting and disease-fighting properties.

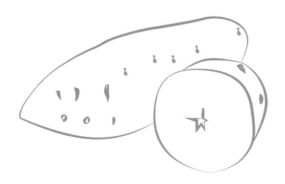

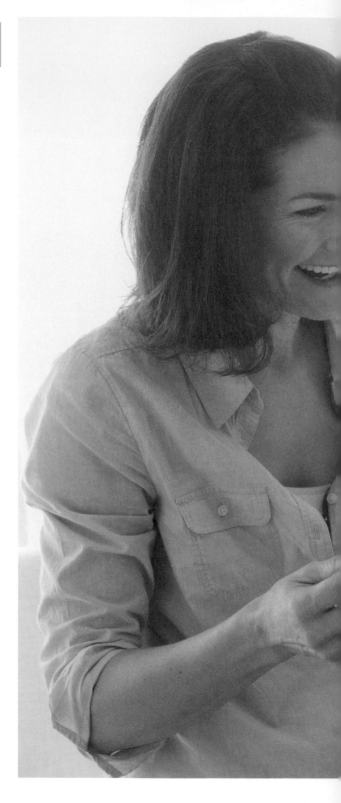

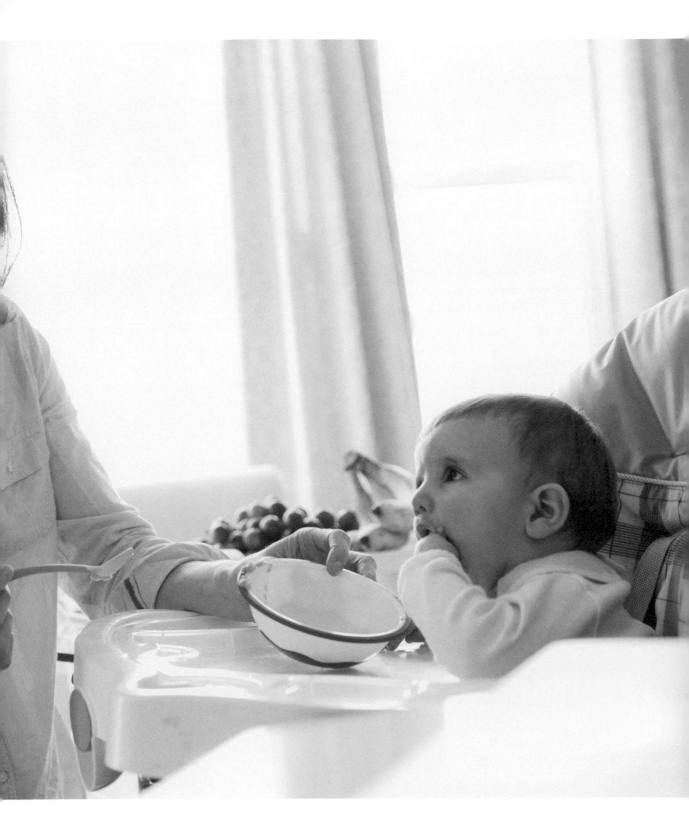

BEATING FATIGUE

There are a number of clever tips for beating the constant fatigue associated with caring for a baby and young children, but number one is to ditch the sugar. As tempting as a cup of sugary tea and a biscuit or a can of fizzy drink may seem, they are just setting your body off into a vicious cycle of short-lived satisfaction, followed by low energy, hunger pangs and craving for more sugar, and the whole cycle starts again. Once you go into the low-energy stage you are likely to feel lethargic, more irritable or less able to concentrate. You might laugh this off as baby brain – and we have all experienced that – but sugar cravings could really be affecting your mood and energy levels.

Cutting out sugar doesn't mean you are on a diet – new mums have to eat and not diet! Concentrate on restoring good health first and there is time to think about active weight loss later as your baby is coming up to a year. In fact, a healthy balanced diet will aid natural, slow weight loss as it will give you more energy to be active, help you sleep better, and prevent weight gain around the tummy that comes from eating too much sugar, which is notoriously hard to shift once it gets there.

HEALTHY SNACK IDEAS

SNACKS FROM THE FRIDGE	SNACKS OUT AND ABOUT
Cubes of pear and cheese	Courgette muffins (see page 183) or Pepper and goat's cheese muffins (see page 185)
Hummus, apple and avocado wrap (see page 118) with cucumber dippers	Cheese and apple scones (see page 180)
Wholegrain toast fingers with soft cheese and chopped dates	Carrot and cinnamon cupcakes (see page 190)
Sardine dip on oatcakes (see page 119)	Quinoa and blueberry pancakes (see page 188)
Slices of apple with nut butter (see page 103)	Apple and blackberry loaf (see page 191)
Quick guacamole (see page 177) with slices of tomato	Fruity flapjacks (see page 196)

To avoid falling into the sugar trap, have plenty of healthy snacks at home or to hand for when you feel hungry. If you try not to eat, you're more likely to succumb to a big sugar-laden treat when you see it. Grabbing a handful or two of almonds can really offset the desire for a doughnut. If you really fancy something sweet, try one of the refined-sugar-free recipes from the final chapter of this book. They are all designed to have a balance of protein, good carbs and healthy fats, which means they are satisfying and can help you to feel fuller for longer. They contain ingredients that are rich in vitamins, minerals and fibre and that won't disrupt your blood-sugar levels.

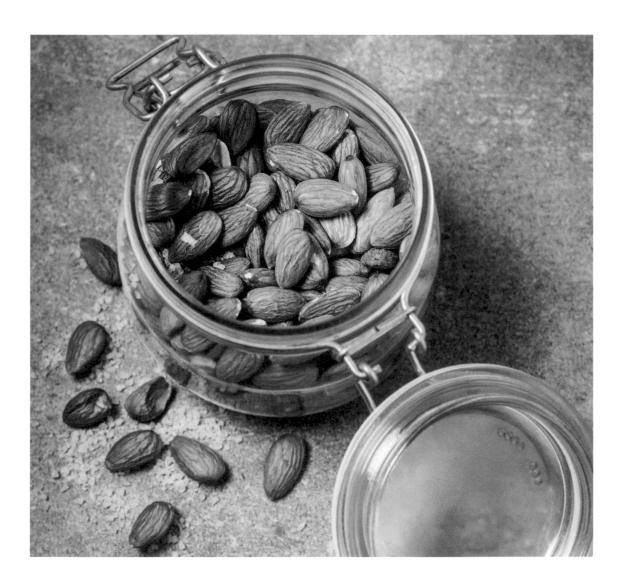

STAYING HYDRATED

Sipping on water regularly throughout the day is the best way to keep well hydrated. Just a drop in your body water levels of 2 per cent – not enough to make you feel thirsty – can still have the effect of making you feel tired and listless. Drinking water boosts energy levels and helps you concentrate, whereas chronic dehydration can cause headaches, a dry mouth and disrupts sleep. Get into the habit of drinking more water and you'll find that this simple thing can impact hugely on your physical and mental abilities. Carry a large bottle of water with you in your changing bag; one with a sports top is useful as you don't need two hands to open it. Tap water, preferably filtered, is fine. If you find plain water too boring, liven it up with a few sprigs of fresh mint, slices of lime, lemon and orange, or a few drops of vanilla extract.

If you are still breastfeeding, remember you need extra water to replace that lost in making breast milk. The advice is to always have a large glass of water to drink whilst you feed, but that doesn't rule out other healthy drinks. Tea (herbal or otherwise) and coffee are fine, although you may want to avoid caffeine if you are hoping to grab some sleep later, and be careful of hot liquids around your baby. A milky drink during a night feed may help you get off to sleep and has the added benefit of providing plenty of calcium. If you're getting bored of water try coconut water, vegetable juices, diluted pure fruit juice or green smoothies.

RESTORING ENERGY LEVELS

Protein is important for feeling energised, and good-quality proteins included at each meal will give you all the essential amino acids your body needs for the growth and repair of cells. Although chicken, fish and yogurt are obvious choices, don't overlook the protein in wholegrains, pulses, nuts and seeds.

Omega-3 fats are important for maintaining energy levels since they have a vital role in energy production as well as being crucial for good mental health, brain function and immunity, which if compromised can leave you feeling lethargic and run-down.

Oily fish such as salmon, mackerel and sardines are the richest source of omega-3 fatty acids, but they are also found in wholegrains, nuts, seeds and oils, in particular flaxseed and walnuts.

One of the first nutrients to suffer when you don't eat properly is iron. In addition, your iron stores may be depleted if you have experienced some heavy bleeding after having your baby. Iron is needed for the production of healthy red blood cells that carry oxygen around the body, so a lack of iron can leave you feeling constantly fatigued.

Red unprocessed meats provide iron in a form that is easily absorbed by the body, so if you like meat try a few of the easy slow-cook stews and tagines. If you're not keen on red meat, you can get iron from wholegrains, green leafy veg such as spinach and cabbage, kidney beans, chickpeas, nuts and dried fruit. NB, avoid eating handfuls of dried fruit between

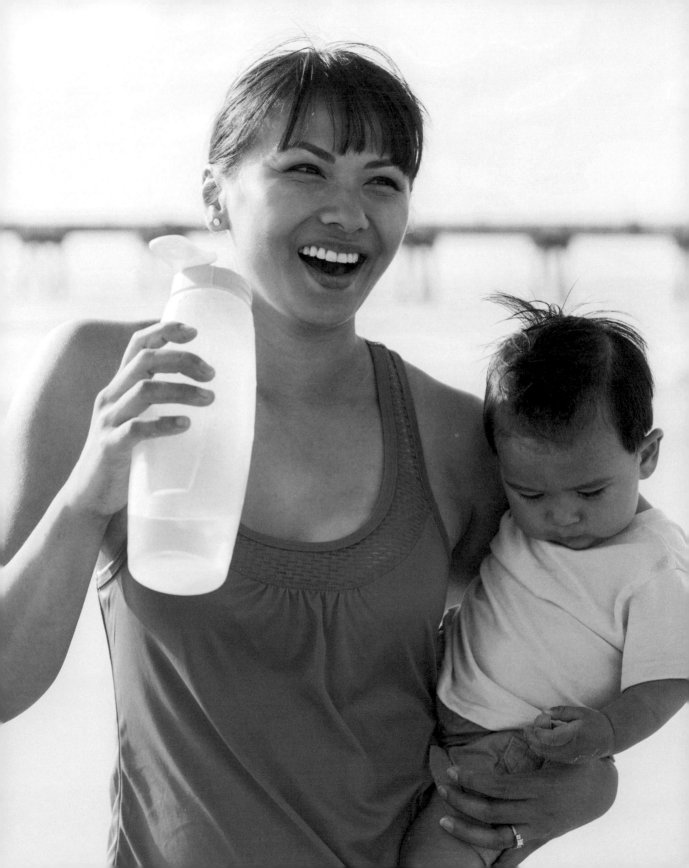

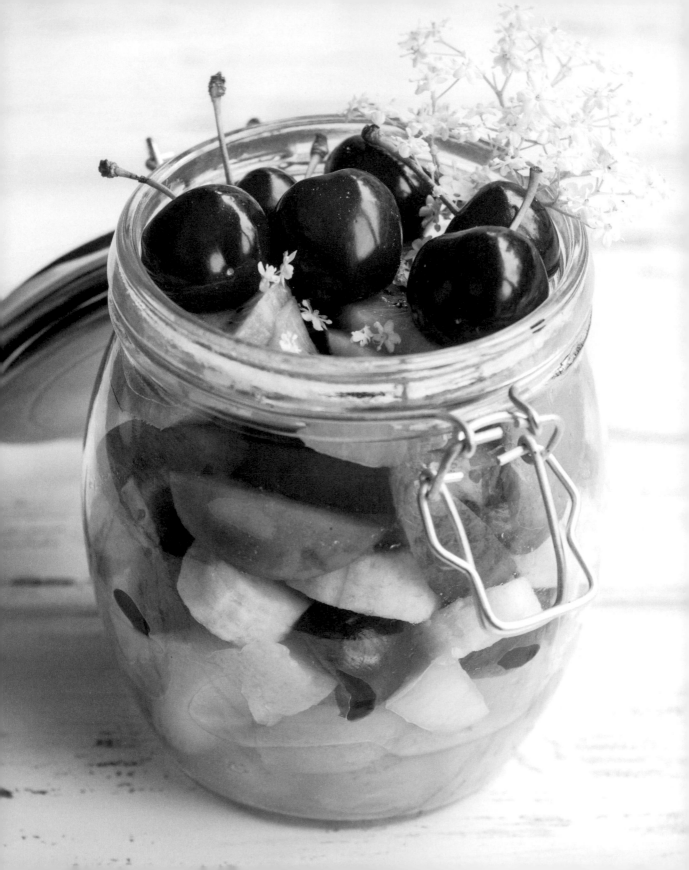

meals: eating too many will disrupt blood-sugar levels. Instead, incorporate them into balanced meals (see the Spicy turkey and apricot meatballs on page 130), as the presence of other nutrients including protein, vitamin C and beta-carotene helps the absorption of iron into the body.

IMPROVING YOUR MOOD

Fluctuations in blood-sugar levels are associated with changes in mood and energy, and are affected by what we eat. After eating sugary foods or refined carbs such as white bread, pasta and breakfast cereals, blood-sugar levels can rise rapidly, which may cause feelings of stress and anxiety, only to crash soon after, which can then leave you feeling lethargic and in a low mood. Blood-sugar crashes can also cause cravings and an uncontrollable appetite.

Choosing foods that have a low GI means they release their energy slowly into the bloodstream and stop blood-sugar levels from dipping. The slow release of energy keeps blood-sugar levels steady and maintains a more balanced, calm mood.
Some examples:

MEDIUM-GI FOODS
- Grapes
- Fresh dates
- Kiwi fruit
- Corn
- Porridge
- Wholegrain
- Oranges
- Mangoes
- Raw carrots
- Peas
- Oatmeal
- Rye bread (including pumpernickel) and brown Basmati rice

LOW-GI FOODS
- Apples
- Peaches
- Plums
- Dried apricots
- Green leafy vegetables
- Pears
- Grapefruits
- Cherries
- Avocados
- Lentils
- Beans and soya products

SLEEPING WELL

Eating well can also improve your sleep. Understandably you may be thinking 'what sleep?!' But as you are likely to be woken up during the night, it's even more important that the sleep you do have is of a good quality to help you feel as rested and refreshed as you can. Foods such as seeds, nuts, beans and pulses contain substances that help to balance hormones and promote the production of ones we need for sleep. Particularly important for sleep is the hormone melatonin which plays a key role in synchronizing circadian rhythms and helps regulate the sleep-wake cycle. Melatonin is found in fruits and veg including tomatoes, cherries, grapes and walnuts are also a good source.

HEALTHY CHOICES

This is my list of 'must have' foods to keep you energised, healthy, happy and well:

FOOD: WHOLEGRAIN BASMATI
Why eat it: Low GI, meaning energy is released slowly, keeping blood-sugar levels steady and maintaining a more balanced, calm mood. Wholegrain basmati also provides vitamins and minerals that are important for good mental health.
What to do with it: Serve with stews, casseroles, tagines and use in pilaffs and kedgeree.

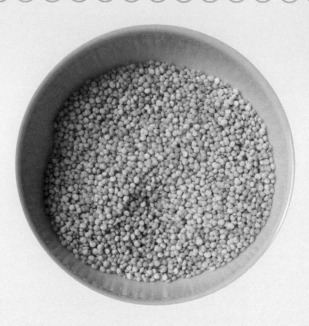

FOOD: QUINOA
Why eat it: Quinoa provides a mix of complex carbohydrate and fibre which helps to maintain stable blood-sugar levels as well as a higher amount of protein, compared with most grains, which can help to control appetite and reduce cravings for sugary and fatty snacks between meals. Feeling more in control of your appetite can reduce stress levels and help you make healthier choices at mealtimes.
What to do with it: Use in salads and add to soups and stews. It also blends well with other grains such as oats in porridge and rice in risottos.

FOOD: PUMPKIN SEEDS
Why eat it: These seeds provide tryptophan, which is an amino acid that is needed to make several important hormones, including the mood-regulating neurotransmitter serotonin. Serotonin plays a role in fighting anxiety, promoting good moods and producing the sleep hormone melatonin. Tryptophan also helps the body to produce important B-vitamin niacin, which is needed for good mental health and to prevent depression.
What to do with it: Roast your own pumpkin seeds and keep in an airtight container and use to sprinkle on to salads, breakfast cereals and porridge, stir into yogurts, and use in baking.

FOOD: CHIA SEEDS

Why eat it: Chia seed is rich in protein and in particular tryptophan, an amino acid that promotes good mood, good sleep and a sense of calm. They are also rich in fibre, potassium, calcium, iron, phosphorus and manganese. Just 1 tbsp (15g) of chia seeds contains 5g of fibre. So adding a tablespoon of chia seeds to your breakfast (cereals, smoothies, juices, etc.) is a great way to increase your fibre intake and stabilise blood-sugar levels.

What to do with it: Soak chia seeds in coconut water or yogurt overnight and then mix with fruit for a nutritious breakfast.

FOOD: CHICKPEAS

Why eat it: Chickpeas contain substances known as phytoestrogens, which can help to balance hormones including testosterone. When the level of this hormone rises, mood can be affected and increase feelings of stress and anxiety. The phytoestrogens help to stimulate the production of another hormone, which binds testosterone and prevents excess levels circulating in the blood. Chickpeas also contain plenty of fibre, which can prevent fluctuations in blood-sugar levels.

What to do with it: Add to salads, soups and stews and use to make hummus.

FOOD: COCONUT

Why eat it: Coconut flesh is high in protein and fibre and is a great source of a healthier type of saturated fat. The saturated fat in coconut oil supports the thyroid gland and the nervous system, both of which are important for maintaining energy levels and a positive mood.

What to do with it: Add to curries and grate into yogurt.

FOOD: PAK CHOI/SPINACH/KALE

Why eat it: Energy, appetite, mood, weight and body temperature are all governed by hormones produced by the thyroid gland. Thyroid hormones affect metabolism, and an imbalance can produce a wide variety of symptoms: an underactive thyroid can cause weight

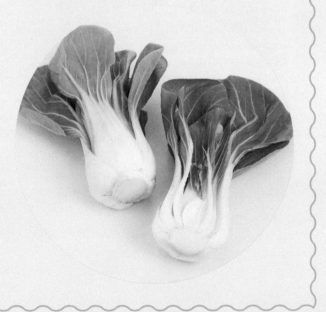

gain, put you in a low mood and make you feel sluggish and cold all the time. Pak choi contains important vitamins including vitamins A, C and E – needed for the healthy production of thyroid hormones.

What to do with it: Use in stir-fries and soups.

FOOD: **BEANS**

Why eat it: Including beans such as kidney, pinto and black-eyed beans in the diet helps to reduce the amount of insulin needed after eating. Insulin is released to regulate blood-sugar levels, but when too much is produced, mood and energy levels can be negatively affected. The fibre, protein and complex carbs in beans reduce the insulin response.

What to do with it: Replace half the quantity of red meat in dishes such as bolognaise, cottage pie or chilli con carne with beans.

FOOD: **CHICKEN/TURKEY**

Why eat it: Chicken and turkey provides vitamin B_6, which is needed for the production of the sleep hormone melatonin that aids good sleep patterns and improves mood. It also provides chromium, a trace element that can help the body use insulin more effectively and so improve energy levels. Eating more turkey breast is a good way to increase your intake of the amino acid tryptophan. Turkey also contains another amino acid, tyrosine, which can help reduce symptoms of depression as well as help you avoid feeling the blues in the first place. Tyrosine is used to make the hormone adrenaline – low levels of which have been associated with depression.

What to do with it: Use in wraps and pitta pockets. Use turkey mince instead of beef mince in cottage pie or chilli.

FOOD: **AVOCADO**

Why eat it: Avocados provide a source of tryptophan, which is converted into serotonin, promoting happiness and relaxation. They also contain omega-3 fatty acids which are important in reducing the risk of depression.

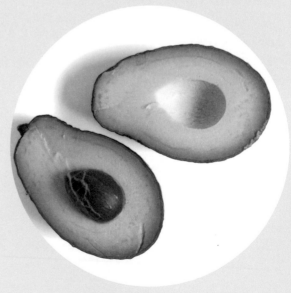

What to do with it: Slice or mash and add to pittas instead of mayonnaise, or use in salads, as a healthy snack on its own, or in cooking (you can make a delicious sugar-free chocolate mousse with it!).

FOOD: BLUEBERRIES

Why eat it: Blueberries are a natural feel-good food. They contain large amounts of vitamins and antioxidants that can help you feel more energetic and promote a healthier mood.

What to do with it: Throw into porridge, blend with yogurt to make smoothies, enjoy them on their own, or use them in baking.

FOOD: BANANAS

Why eat it: Bananas contain tryptophan and also vitamins A, B_6 and C, fibre, potassium, phosphorous, iron and carbohydrate. Carbs aid in the absorption of tryptophan in the brain, and vitamin B_6 helps convert the tryptophan into the mood-lifting hormone serotonin. This helps to boost your mood and also aids good sleep.

What to do with it: Slice on to wholemeal toast spread with nut butter, use in smoothies, eat raw, or use them in baking.

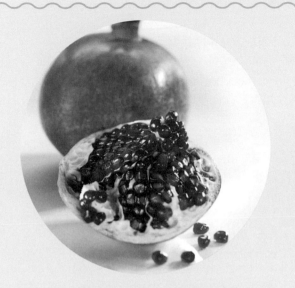

FOOD: POMEGRANATES

Why eat it: The phytochemicals found in pomegranates stimulate the oestrogen and serotonin receptors in the body, which in turn then helps to boost mood and lessen feelings of depression.

What to do with it: Add to tagines, couscous and salads, or eat raw.

FOOD: OILY FISH AND WALNUTS

Why eat it: Oily fish and walnuts are rich sources of omega-3 fatty acids. These acids are vital for good mental health, brain function, energy production, oxygen transfer and immunity. Oily fish contain the two long-chain omega-3 fats known as EPA and DHA, which can help to reduce inflammation, high levels of which may be linked to depression. Walnuts provide an essential form of omega fat that can be converted into EPA and DHA.

What to do with it: Oily fish can be used in any number of recipes, but you can also eat good-quality canned ones on their own as a healthy high-protein snack. Sprinkle walnuts on to salads and breakfast cereals, eat them raw as a snack, or use them in baking.

FOOD: OATS
Why eat it: Oats contain plenty of fibre and slow-release carbohydrate to regulate blood-sugar levels and maintain energy levels.
What to do with it: Versatile oats can be used for making porridge, in smoothies, and a huge number of baking recipes, from oatcakes and gluten-free pastry to flapjacks and energy bombs.

FOOD: BRAZIL NUTS
Why eat it: Brazil nuts are the richest source of the mineral selenium, containing 10 times more than the next-richest source. Selenium-rich food helps to combat depression and studies have shown that eating two or three Brazil nuts every day can help to improve mood.
What to do with it: Eat on their own as a snack, chop and sprinkle into yogurt with grated dark chocolate for a healthy dessert, or use in baking.

FOOD: BEETROOT
Why eat it: Beetroots contain a nutrient known as betaine, which can improve the production of the natural mood-enhancing hormone serotonin.
What to do with it: You can buy ready-cooked beetroot in vacuum packs, and these are a quick and easy way to up your beetroot intake. Simply dice and add to salads, or use to make beetroot hummus or brownies.

FOOD: ASPARAGUS/BROCCOLI
Why eat it: Low intakes of the B vitamin folate have been linked to poor mood and risk of depression. These green leafy veg are among the richest sources in our diets.
What to do with it: Serve steamed as a salad, starter or accompaniment with a drizzle of olive oil and a squeeze of lemon juice, use in omelettes and risottos, add to stir-fries, or make 'broccoli couscous' by blitzing some broccoli in a food processor and steaming it with a drop of water for a couple of minutes.

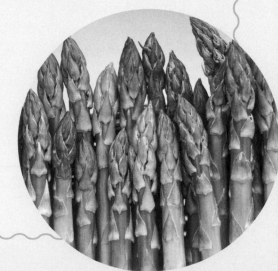

PREPARING FOOD FOR YOUR BABY: SOME PRACTICAL TIPS

It might seem a real effort to start cooking and puréeing food for your baby when there is so much else to do and you haven't slept, but once you start you'll find it is manageable with a bit of strategic planning, and even enjoyable as you get more creative. Choose a time, maybe a weekend morning or a quiet weekday evening, to cook in batches. That way you have the basis of a meal that is ready in minutes for those chaotic days when you feel overwhelmed by all the things you have to do.

BEST COOKING METHODS

Steaming and poaching are the simplest ways of preparing fruit and vegetables. Steaming is a particularly good cooking method since it helps the food to retain more of the nutrients that could otherwise be lost in boiling water. Foods such as apples and pears that need to be puréed should be poached in just a little water to help concentrate the ratio of food to water and avoid making them too slushy. Thin, too-liquid purées will mean your baby will fill up on water at the expense of good nutrition.

Also remember to:
- Cook eggs until the yolk and white are solid
- Cook meats until they are no longer pink in the middle
- Wash and peel fruit and vegetables, such as apples and carrots.

PREPARING THE KITCHEN

Without having to spend a fortune, it is worth investing in a few essential items of equipment and keeping your store cupboard topped up with some key healthy and handy ingredients.

EQUIPMENT YOU WILL NEED

Investing in the right equipment will help simplify the preparation process. A steamer (or steamer basket that sits on top of a pan), a pan, baking tin and a food processor or hand-held blender are all you need to make a wide variety of purées for your baby.

In addition, you will need to be able to safely store it, such as clean, small clip-top pots to store in the refrigerator (you can buy pots that hold just a couple of tablespoonfuls of purée). If you intend to freeze portions (which is highly recommended), you'll need ice-cube trays with a lid, and freezer bags. Once they get older, you can freeze larger portions in special baby food trays with lids that hold larger amounts.

There is nothing more frustrating when you have planned to cook and find you have run out of one of the store cupboard basics like a spice or a jar of mustard. And it's good to know that there is nothing nutritionally inferior with tinned tomatoes or frozen fruit and veg. So do one big shop and stock your cupboard well so it won't thwart your efforts to get in the kitchen and cook. In the long term it's not expensive, as your supplies will happily sit in your cupboard and freezer for months.

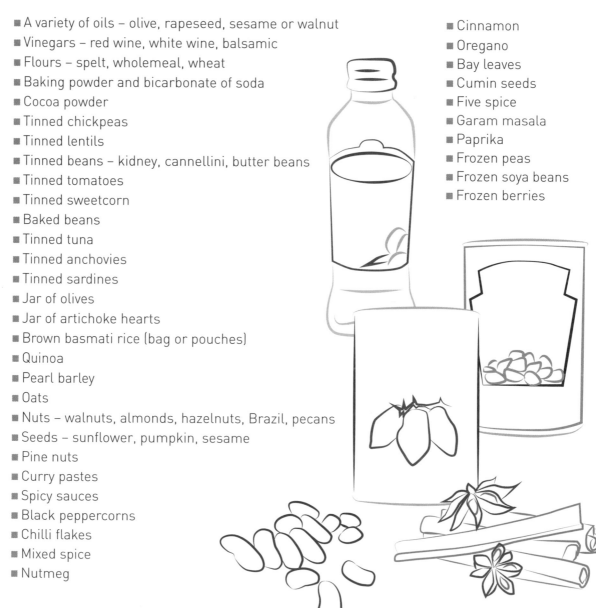

- A variety of oils – olive, rapeseed, sesame or walnut
- Vinegars – red wine, white wine, balsamic
- Flours – spelt, wholemeal, wheat
- Baking powder and bicarbonate of soda
- Cocoa powder
- Tinned chickpeas
- Tinned lentils
- Tinned beans – kidney, cannellini, butter beans
- Tinned tomatoes
- Tinned sweetcorn
- Baked beans
- Tinned tuna
- Tinned anchovies
- Tinned sardines
- Jar of olives
- Jar of artichoke hearts
- Brown basmati rice (bag or pouches)
- Quinoa
- Pearl barley
- Oats
- Nuts – walnuts, almonds, hazelnuts, Brazil, pecans
- Seeds – sunflower, pumpkin, sesame
- Pine nuts
- Curry pastes
- Spicy sauces
- Black peppercorns
- Chilli flakes
- Mixed spice
- Nutmeg

- Cinnamon
- Oregano
- Bay leaves
- Cumin seeds
- Five spice
- Garam masala
- Paprika
- Frozen peas
- Frozen soya beans
- Frozen berries

STORING YOUR BABY'S FOOD

As a general rule, freshly cooked food will keep up to 3 days in the fridge and for up to three months in the freezer. When you have made a batch of purées, keep a few in the fridge and freeze the rest. Let the food cool to room temperature before you put it in the fridge or freezer.

Covered ice-cube trays are ideal for freezing baby-sized portions of purée. Fill a few trays with a batch of purée and freeze just as you would ice cubes. Once frozen, transfer them to a freezer bag, this way they take up less room and you can use your trays for another purée batch. Label everything you freeze with the contents and the date as you may not recognise it a few weeks later.

THAWING, REHEATING AND TRANSPORTING YOUR BABY'S FOOD

Both thawing and reheating can promote the growth of bacteria, so follow these simple guidelines to keep your baby's food safe:

■ If you will not be reheating thawed purée (ie if you are mixing some apple purée into some yogurt), you should thaw it in the fridge and use it as soon as it is completely defrosted. To bring purées from the fridge to room temperature, leave it out, covered for 15–20 minutes. Do not let your baby's food sit out in the kitchen for more than an hour, or 30 minutes in hot weather.

■ The best way to reheat purées is in a pan over a low to medium heat. Be aware that microwaving is not recommended as this can cause uneven heating and hot spots, which could burn your baby's mouth. If you do use a microwave, make sure you stir well half way through and then leave to stand for a few minutes and then stir again and taste yourself. When reheating baby food, make sure it's piping hot throughout – you should be able to see steam coming out. Don't reheat your baby's food more than once.

■ Let food cool down before you give it to your baby and always check the temperature before feeding. To do this, simply dab a tiny bit of food on the inside of your wrist or back of your hand to see if it's a comfortable temperature before giving it to him.

■ Don't be tempted to give food to your baby again after a few hours, or to refreeze leftovers, since bacteria levels may be too high. You could eat it yourself, but do be aware that grazing on your baby's (and children's) leftovers is an easy way for the calories to creep up.

■ If you are going out and want to take some home-made food with you, heat it up as normal, then place it straight into a sterilised clip-top container and seal it shut so no bacteria can enter.

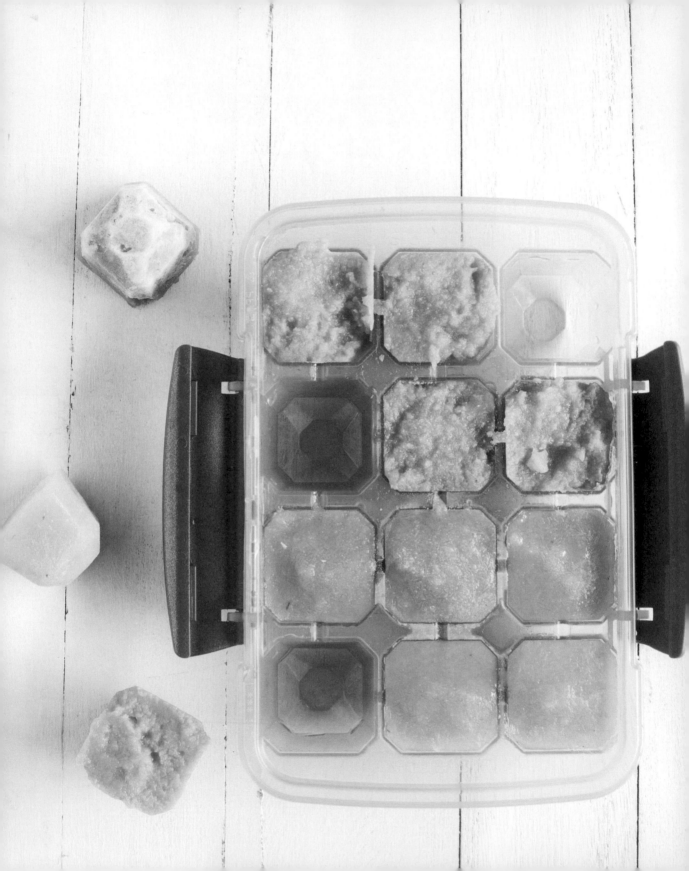

HOW TO STERILISE BABY FEEDING EQUIPMENT

There are several ways you can sterilise your baby's feeding equipment. These include using a cold water sterilising solution, by steam sterilising, or boiling.

Before sterilising, always clean the feeding item, be it a bottle and teat or a bowl in hot, soapy water as soon as possible after using and use a bottlebrush for bottles (and only use it for the bottles). Then rinse all your equipment in clean, cold running water before sterilising.

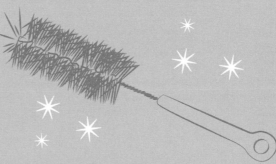

COLD WATER STERILISING SOLUTION
- Change the sterilising solution every 24 hours.

- Leave feeding equipment in the sterilising solution for at least 30 minutes.

- Make sure there is no air trapped in the bottles or teats when putting them in the sterilising solution.

- Keep all the equipment under the solution with a floating cover.

STEAM STERILISING
(Electric steriliser or microwave)
- It's important to follow the manufacturer's instructions, as there are several different types of sterilisers.

- Make sure the openings of the bottles and teats are facing downwards in the steriliser.

- Manufacturers will give guidelines on how long you can leave equipment that you are not using immediately (straight after sterilising) before it needs to be resterilised.

STERILISING BY BOILING
- Make sure that whatever you sterilise in this way is safe to boil.

- Boil the feeding equipment in water for at least 10 minutes, making sure that all items stay under the water's surface.

- Teats tend to get damaged faster with this method so check regularly that teats and bottles are not torn, cracked or damaged.

- Wash your hands thoroughly. Clean and disinfect the surface where you will put together the bottle and teat.

- It's best to remove the bottles just before they are used.

- If the bottles are not being used immediately, they should be put together fully with the teat and lid in place. This is to prevent the inside of the sterilised bottle from being contaminated, along with the inside and outside of the teat.

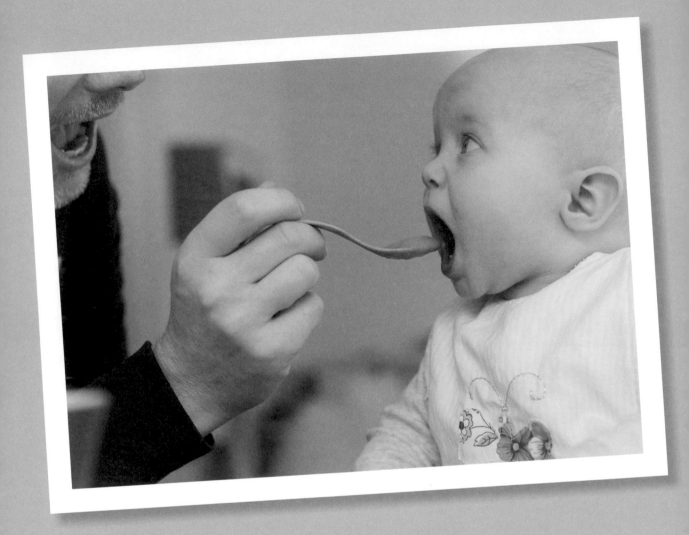
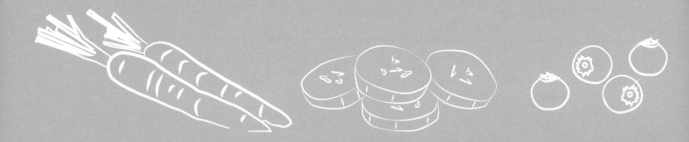

STAGE 1
PURÉES

So, the time has come and you are ready to
start offering your baby their first tastes of food.
These are the simplest and easiest recipes
that your baby will love and you can share.

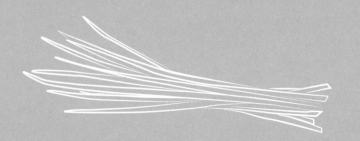

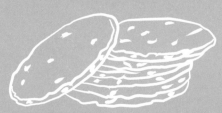

BABY AVOCADO PURÉE
YOU CHICKEN & AVOCADO WRAP

Avocados are one of the best starting foods to offer your baby. They contain healthy unsaturated fats that are needed for brain and cognitive development and for the growth of the nervous system, and they have a mild, not-too-sweet taste and a natural creamy consistency that can be easily digested by your baby's still-developing gut. For you, they are a great source of vitamin E, a powerful antioxidant that boosts the immune system and is important for keeping skin healthy. The beneficial fats they provide help to prevent inflammation in the body and assist in the absorption of other vitamins and antioxidants from your food.

Preparation time: 10 mins
Cooking time: 0 mins

TO PREPARE
One ripe avocado

FOR BABY
3 avocado slices
2 tbsp (30ml) of your baby's usual milk

FOR YOU
Serves 1
1 spring onion
The remaining unmashed avocado
1 tomato
1 cooked chicken breast
1 tbsp (15ml) crème fraîche, sour cream or plain Greek yogurt
A sprinkle of hot chilli sauce (optional)
1 soft wholemeal seeded tortilla

This is a quick and easy lunch, great for those times when you're feeling tempted just to open a packet of biscuits. It uses pre-cooked chicken (see 'Cook Ahead'), so in just 5 minutes you'll have created a filling, nutritious meal that will keep you going all afternoon and stop that mid-afternoon slump. You can spice it up if you wish with a dash of hot chilli sauce.

Slice the avocado lengthways around the stone and twist apart. Remove the stone and score through the flesh lengthways. Use the tip of the knife to gently run along the inside of the skin; the slices of avocado should fall away.

FOR BABY AVOCADO PURÉE
Roughly chop the avocado slices and place in a small bowl. Mash with a fork or the back of a spoon to form a creamy paste. Add the milk and stir well to achieve a smooth, runny consistency. Serve immediately, since it will quickly go brown.

FOR YOU CHICKEN AND AVOCADO WRAP
Use scissors to snip the spring onion into a bowl. Roughly chop the avocado, tomato and chicken breast and add them to the spring onion. Mix in the crème fraîche, sour cream or Greek yogurt and sprinkle with the chilli sauce, if using. Spread the filling along the middle of the tortilla and roll it up to form a wrap, tucking in the tortilla at each end. Slice in half.

COOK AHEAD
I cook a batch of chicken breasts at the beginning of the week so I have some on standby in the fridge to make a nutritious, sustaining snack, or you can buy cooked chicken breasts at the supermarket.

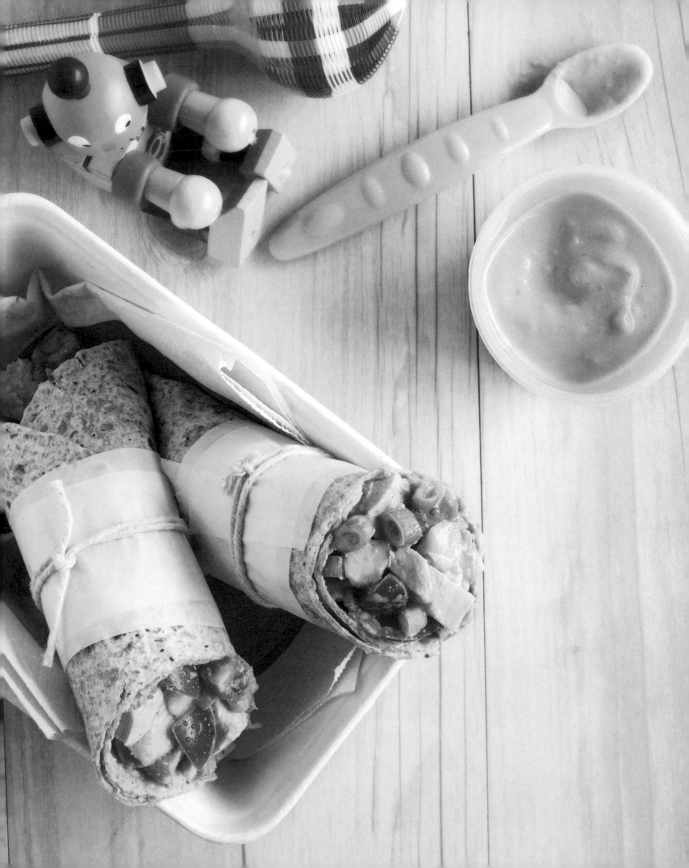

BABY BANANA PURÉE
YOU BROWN RICE & QUINOA BANANA SMOOTHIE

Bananas are another tried-and-tested first food for your baby to sample. They are easily digested and have a creamy taste and a natural sweetness that will tempt your baby to eat solids. Bananas are often wrongly thought of as being 'high in sugar'. In fact, while they do contain some fructose (natural fruit sugar), they also contain fibres called pectins that give bananas a low GI (glycaemic index) because they slow the absorption of fructose into the bloodstream. Bananas also contain a type of carbohydrate that is typically not broken down by enzymes in the digestive tract. Instead, they move along until they reach the lower intestine and get metabolised by bacteria. This is a crucial process in new babies that helps to maintain the balance of 'friendly' bacteria to support healthy digestion, boost immunity and help to prevent risk of infections. Bananas are a good source of potassium, an essential mineral for maintaining normal blood pressure and heart function. They also contain small amounts of substances called sterols, which have the ability to block the absorption of dietary cholesterol and so help to maintain healthy blood-cholesterol levels.

Preparation time: 5 mins
Cooking time: 2 mins

TO PREPARE
One ripe bananna

FOR BABY
3 banana chunks

2 tbsp (30ml) of your baby's usual milk

FOR YOU
Serves 1

2 tbsp (30ml) cooked brown basmati rice and quinoa

The remaining unmashed banana

½ tsp (2.5ml) ground cinnamon

200ml almond or other milk

1 tbsp (15ml) plain Greek yogurt

A drizzle of honey (optional)

A handful of flaked almonds

This is a great smoothie for those times when you really want something sweet, satisfying the craving without having disastrous effects on your blood-sugar levels. Cinnamon can help to regulate insulin levels so use it whenever you can. I've included almond milk here just because it adds a nice nutty flavour, but your regular milk is fine. You can add a dollop of plain Greek yogurt for extra creaminess but don't worry if you don't have it to hand – the smoothie is still delicious without it.

Peel and roughly chop a medium-sized banana.

FOR BABY BANANA PURÉE
Put the banana chunks in a small bowl and mash with a fork or the back of a spoon to form a creamy paste. Add the milk and stir well to achieve a smooth, runny consistency. Serve immediately, since it will quickly go brown.

FOR YOU BROWN RICE & QUINOA BANANA SMOOTHIE
Put the rice and quinoa in a blender, then add the banana, cinnamon, milk and yogurt and whizz together. Transfer to a glass, drizzle in the honey, if using, and sprinkle over the almonds.

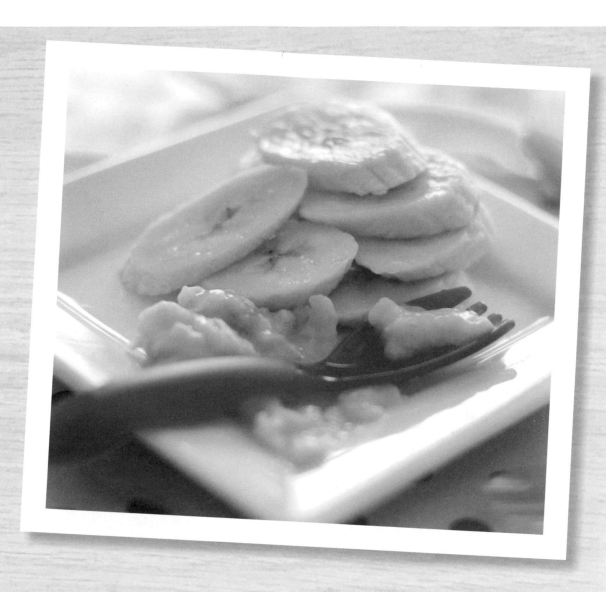

REHEATING RICE

Microwave pouches are by far the most convenient way to cook brown rice and quinoa; simply follow the instructions on the packet. Having taken what you need for the smoothie, you can store the remaining rice in the pouch for a couple of days so long as it is sealed securely and stored in the fridge until you need it. When ready to eat, transfer the leftover rice and quinoa from the pouch into a pan and stir-fry it with a little oil. Make sure the rice is piping hot and thoroughly heated before you eat it; don't use it cold in another smoothie, as it really does need to be thoroughly reheated before consumption.

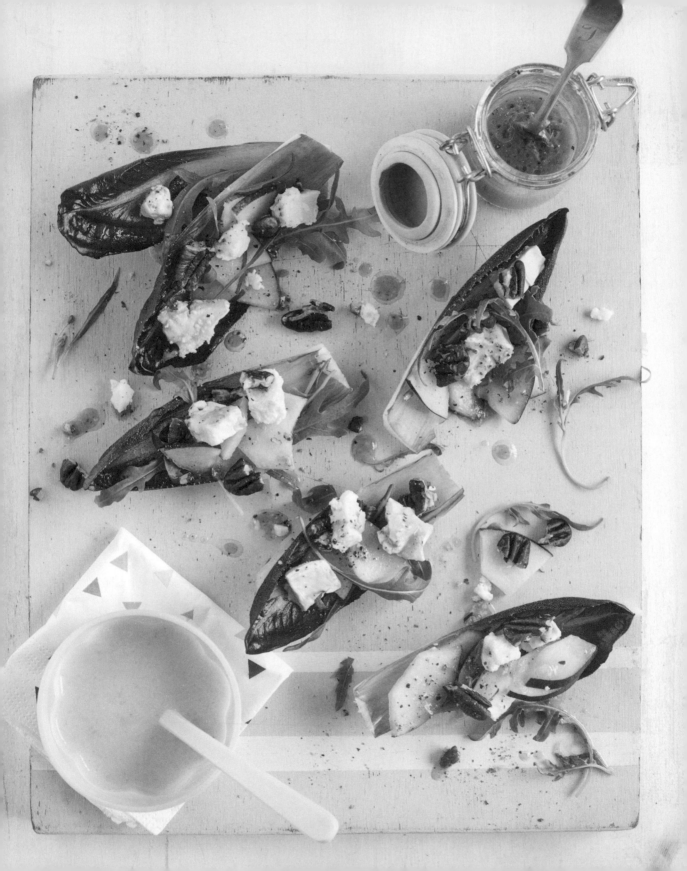

BABY PEAR PURÉE
YOU CHICORY BOATS WITH PEAR & PECANS

Pears are a perfect introduction to solids for your baby because they are considered to be one of the most readily digestible and hypoallergenic foods, meaning they are less likely to cause a nasty reaction such as a rash or an upset tummy the first time they are eaten. Pears contain flavanoids that can improve insulin sensitivity and so reduce the risk of developing type 2 diabetes. Pears also contain other phytonutrients that have antioxidant, anti-inflammatory and anti-cancer properties.

Preparation time: 10 mins
Cooking time: 5-8 mins

TO PREPARE
A bag of 6 pears

FOR BABY
3 cubes frozen pear purée, thawed, or 3 tbsp (45ml) pear purée

2 tbsp (30ml) of your baby's usual milk

1 tsp (5ml) baby rice flakes (optional)

FOR YOU
Serves 2
The remaining raw pear

50g goat's cheese

1 head of red chicory

A large handful of rocket leaves

2 tbsp (30ml) pecan nuts

1 tbsp (15ml) pear purée

2 tbsp (30ml) sherry or red wine vinegar

1 tbsp (15ml) olive or rapeseed oil

Salt and ground black pepper

Chicory gives a mildly peppery background flavour that is nicely balanced by the natural sweetness of the pear and the creaminess of the cheese. You can use different salad leaves, but one advantage of chicory is that the leaves can be held in one hand, leaving your other hand free.

Peel five of the pears, then cut them into quarters and remove the cores. Pour water to a depth of 2.5cm into a pan and bring to the boil. Place the pear quarters into a steamer basket or glass bowl and cover with a lid. Steam over the water for 5–8 minutes, until tender (this will depend on ripeness). Allow to cool, then transfer to a food processor or blender. Whizz until smooth.

If you want to use a microwave, place the pear quarters in a suitable bowl with a drop of water, cover and microwave on High for 2 minutes. Check the pears, then microwave for a further 1–2 minutes, or until the pears are soft.

You can store the pear purée in an airtight container in the fridge for up to three days. Alternatively, fill ice-cube trays with the mixture and freeze for up to a month.

FOR BABY PEAR PURÉE
Mix together the pear purée and milk in a bowl until you achieve a smooth, runny consistency. For a slightly thicker texture, reduce the amount of milk you add, or stir in a spoonful of baby rice flakes. The latter will make the mixture more sustaining.

FOR YOU CHICORY BOATS WITH PEAR & PECANS
Halve the pear, then remove the core and finely slice the flesh. Cube the cheese.

Trim away the chicory stalk ends and discard any limp or tired outer leaves. Carefully separate the leaves and divide them between two serving plates. To the inside of each chicory-leaf 'boat', add a few rocket leaves, a slice of pear, a cube of cheese and a sprinkle of pecan nuts.

Make a dressing by placing the pear purée, vinegar and oil into a bowl. Season with a pinch of salt and plenty of ground black pepper and whisk or shake together. Drizzle over the chicory leaves.

BABY APPLE PURÉE
YOU APPLE, FETA & WALNUT SALAD

Choose sweet-tasting apples for your baby's purée, such as Golden Delicious, Pink Lady or Gala varieties. Although they taste like it, they are not actually high in sugar. Apples contain phytonutrients that can help to keep blood-sugar levels even and prevent spikes. They also contain a substance called quercitin that stops enzymes from breaking down complex carbohydrates into simple sugars that would otherwise cause a sugar rush. In addition, apples are packed with pectin fibre that can help to maintain healthy levels of fat in the blood and also keep your appetite in check and prevent hunger pangs between meals.

Preparation time: 10 mins
Cooking time: 10-12 mins

TO PREPARE
A bag of 6 apples

FOR BABY
3 cubes frozen apple purée, thawed, or 3 tbsp (45ml) apple purée

2 tbsp (30ml) of your baby's usual milk

A pinch of cinnamon (optional)

FOR YOU
Serves 1
The remaining 1 raw apple

2 large handfuls of baby spinach leaves or watercress

1 spring onion

1 tbsp (15ml) chopped walnut pieces

1 tbsp (15ml) dried cranberries

30g feta cheese

1 tbsp (15ml) apple purée

2 tbsp (30ml) cider vinegar

1 tbsp (15ml) olive or rapeseed oil

Salt and ground black pepper

The partnership of apple and feta makes a crisp and tangy salad, perfect for those days when you need a dish to help you feel energised. The feta is a good source of protein and calcium, which you need more of if you are still breastfeeding. The walnuts and cranberries add crunch and a touch of sweetness but you can use whichever nuts and dried fruit you have in the cupboard.

Peel five of the apples, then cut them into quarters and remove the cores. Pour water to a depth of 2.5cm into a pan and bring to the boil. Place the apple quarters into a steamer basket or glass bowl and cover with a lid. Steam over the water for 10–12 minutes, until tender. Allow to cool, then transfer to a food processor or blender. Whizz until smooth.

If you want to use a microwave, place the apple quarters in a suitable bowl with a drop of water, cover and microwave on High for 2 minutes. Check the apples, and microwave for a further 2–3 minutes, or until the apples are soft. This will vary a little depending upon the variety.

You can store the apple purée in an airtight container in the fridge for up to 3 days. Alternatively, fill ice-cube trays with the mixture and freeze for up to a month.

FOR BABY APPLE PURÉE
Mix together the apple purée and milk in a bowl until you achieve a smooth, runny consistency. You could try adding a pinch of cinnamon for extra flavour.

FOR YOU APPLE, FETA & WALNUT SALAD
Halve the remaining apple, then remove the core and thinly slice. Place the spinach leaves in a large serving bowl. Use scissors to snip the spring onion and add to the spinach with the slices of apple. Toss in the walnuts and cranberries and crumble over the feta.

Make a dressing by placing the apple purée, vinegar and oil into a bowl or a clean jar. Season with a pinch of salt and plenty of ground black pepper and whisk or shake together. Drizzle over the salad and serve.

BABY SWEET POTATO PURÉE

YOU BAKED SWEET POTATO WITH SPICY CHICKPEAS

Sweet potatoes make a great staple for your baby as they are packed with important vitamins needed to support her growth. They are rich in beta-carotene (a form of vitamin A), which is needed for healthy eyesight. They also provide vitamin C and minerals such as copper (vital for the healthy functioning of the organs as well metabolic processes) and iron. Their natural sweetness means they are slightly higher in sugar than white potatoes, but don't be put off – the high fibre content gives them a low GI, which means they don't cause a sugar spike. Sweet potatoes also contain substances that have powerful antioxidant effects, protecting cells against damage and inflammation.

Preparation time: 10 mins
Cooking time: 45-50 mins

TO PREPARE
One large sweet potato

FOR BABY
1/3 of the cooked sweet potato

1 cube frozen apple purée, thawed, or 1 tbsp (15ml) fresh apple purée

Your baby's usual milk (optional)

FOR YOU
Serves 1
200g canned chickpeas

A drizzle of olive oil

1 tsp (5ml) cayenne pepper

The remaining cooked sweet potato

1 tomato

1 spring onion

A small pat of butter

For days when you fancy the comfort of something hot, try this yummy baked potato. The chickpeas are a great alternative to baked beans and they take hardly any extra effort to make. They are a good source of protein and fibre and will keep you feeling full and satisfied all afternoon.

Preheat the oven to 200ºC (Gas 6). Scrub the potato, pat it dry and prick it five or six times with a knife. Place it on a baking sheet and bake it in the oven for 45–50 minutes. If you want to use a microwave, place the pricked potato on a plate and microwave on High for 4 minutes. Turn it over, then microwave it for a further 4–6 minutes, checking it frequently, until it is tender (the cooking time will depend upon the size of the sweet potato).

FOR BABY SWEET POTATO PURÉE

When the sweet potato is soft and cooked, slice off about one-third from one end. Scoop out the flesh with a spoon and place it in the bowl with the apple purée, then blend together. You can use a hand-held blender to make a smooth purée and add a little of your baby's usual milk if you want to make it runnier. Or, if you think your baby can manage a thick consistency, just use a fork to mash together the sweet potato and apple.

FOR YOU BAKED SWEET POTATO WITH SPICY CHICKPEAS

Drain the chickpeas, then rinse under running water and dry with kitchen paper. Place them in a bowl, drizzle with olive oil and sprinkle with the cayenne pepper. Toss together to coat well. When there is 15 minutes' baking time remaining for the sweet potato, tip the coated chickpeas on to one side of the baking sheet, away from the sweet potato, and bake the chickpeas and sweet potato together for the remaining cooking time.

Meanwhile, chop the tomato and spring onion and place in a bowl. When the chickpeas and sweet potato are baked, remove your baby's portion from the sweet potato. Slit the remaining part in half, score the flesh with a knife and dot each with a small pat of butter. Mix the chickpeas into the tomato and spring onion, then spoon the mixture over the sweet potato.

BABY BUTTERNUT SQUASH PURÉE

YOU CHICKEN & ROASTED BUTTERNUT SQUASH

Butternut squash is a key provider of carotenoids, including beta-carotene, which can help to keep the eyes healthy, it also has a high pectin content (a type of fibre) and is an essential element in blood sugar regulation throughout the body, making sure that your insulin and glucose levels remain balanced and even. This means that other body organs function well and are kept healthy. Maintaining even blood-sugar levels also help to keep your appetite under control.

Preparation time: 15 mins
Cooking time: 70-80 mins

TO PREPARE
One butternut squash

FOR BABY
½ a butternut squash

Your baby's usual milk

FOR YOU
Serves 2
The remaining butternut squash

2 chicken breasts

Drizzle of olive oil

A pinch of salt and ground black pepper

2 tbsp of hazelnuts

4 handfuls of watercress leaves

10-12 cherry tomatoes

2 spring onions

¼ cucumber

2 tbsp olive or hazelnut oil

2 tbsp good balsamic vinegar

Invite another new mum and her baby for lunch and impress them with this simple delicious salad. Minimal effort is needed here, just a little chopping and shredding, but the caramelised butternut squash gives it the wow factor, adding a lovely sweet flavour that is enhanced by the balsamic dressing.

Preheat the oven to 180°C/Gas 5. Use a heavy, sharp knife to cut the squash in half and then scoop out the seeds (and set aside – see opposite) and discard the fibrous strings.

Put the squash cut side down in a baking tray and add enough water to come 1cm up the sides of the squash. Roast for 50-60 minutes until tender.

FOR BABY BUTTERNUT SQUASH PURÉE
Scoop out the flesh from one half and purée in a food processor until smooth. Transfer 2 tbsp into a bowl and mix with a little of your baby's usual milk if you want a runnier consistency. Use the rest to fill ice cube trays and freeze.

FOR YOU CHICKEN & ROASTED BUTTERNUT SQUASH
When the butternut squash has 20 minutes baking time remaining, place the 2 chicken breasts on a baking sheet, drizzle with a little olive oil, season with a pinch of salt and black pepper and place in the oven.

Once ready, peel the flesh from the other half of the butternut squash and roughly chop into chunks. Place on a baking sheet, drizzle with olive oil and season with a pinch of salt and plenty of black pepper and return to the oven for 10 minutes.

Meanwhile, halve the tomatoes and chop the spring onions and cucumber and place in a bowl with the watercress. Remove the chicken from the oven and slice and add to the bowl.

Once the butternut squash has caramelised, add to the bowl with the hazelnuts, drizzle over the olive oil and balsamic vinegar and lightly toss everything together.

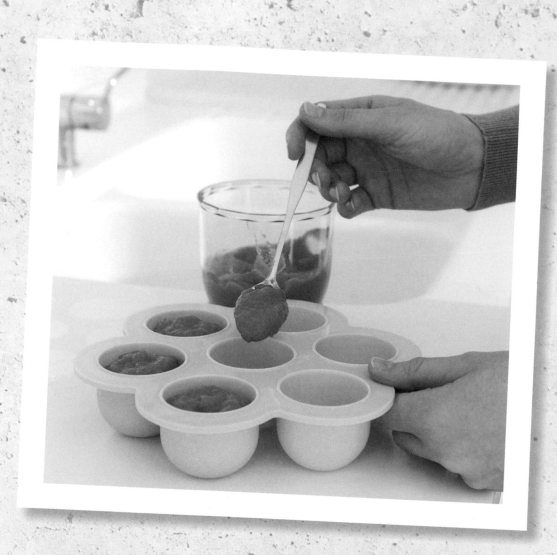

BUTTERNUT SQUASH SEEDS

Seeds from butternut squash and pumpkins make a great snack food for busy mums (they are
not suitable for your baby just yet). They provide protein, healthy fats and plenty of important
minerals such as calcium, zinc and magnesium. They do not disrupt blood sugar levels so
a small handful between meals will satisfy and not have you feeling hungry soon after.
Preheat the oven to 75°C/Gas 1 and place the seeds in a single layer on a baking sheet
and lightly roast them in the oven for 15-20 minutes. By roasting them for a relatively
short time at a low temperature you can help minimise damage to their healthy oils.

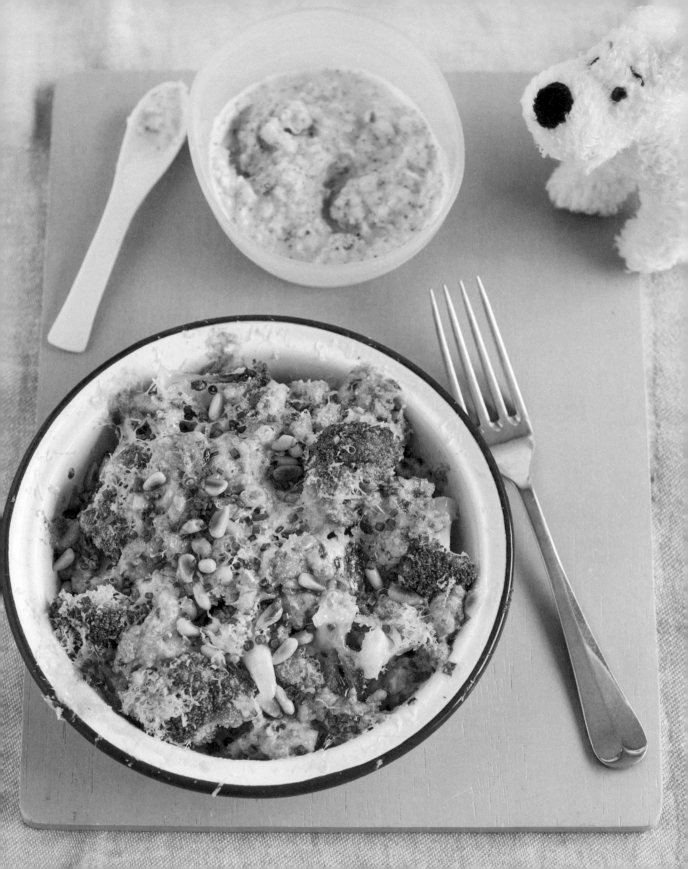

BABY BROCCOLI & PEAR PURÉE
YOU BROCCOLI & PARMESAN GRATIN

It's good to introduce a vegetable with a strong flavour such as broccoli early on to challenge your baby's taste buds and let him experience something different to the mild sweet flavours he has enjoyed so far. To lessen the impact a little, try blending with a little puréed apple or pear. Broccoli is a powerhouse of nutrients providing high amounts of vitamin C and folate as well as vitamins A, K, calcium, fibre, beta-carotene and other antioxidants.

Preparation time: 15 mins
Cooking time: 8-10 mins

TO PREPARE
One head of broccoli

FOR BABY
3 broccoli florets

2 cubes of purée pear

1 tsp creme fraiche

FOR YOU
Serves 1
1 slice of wholemeal or granary bread

2 tbsp crème fraiche

Handful of chives

1 tbsp toasted pine nuts

2 tbsp of finely grated parmesan
(or 1 tbsp each of parmesan and grated Cheddar)

The remaining broccoli

It's good for your baby to watch you eating the same thing as she is, but if you don't fancy tucking into a bowl of plain broccoli try this really simple gratin. The addition of the wholegrain bread and cheese creates a balanced meal providing carbohydrate and protein, while the pine nuts provide healthy fats and vitamin E (you can buy these ready toasted).

Cut the florets of broccoli from the stalk, steam or boil for 8-10 minutes until tender.

FOR BABY BROCCOLI & PEAR PURÉE
While the broccoli is steaming, remove a cube of puréed pear from the freezer and place in a bowl to defrost. When the broccoli is cooked, add three florets to the pear purée and blend using a handheld blender. Don't worry if the pear isn't entirely defrosted, the heat of the broccoli will melt it. Add a teaspoon of crème fraiche and swirl through the purée.

FOR YOU BROCCOLI & PARMESAN GRATIN
Turn on the grill to its highest setting. While the broccoli is steaming, place the slice of bread in a food processor and whizz to create breadcrumbs. Place the breadcrumbs in a bowl and mix in the crème fraiche, chives, pine nuts and 1 tbsp of the cheese.

Place the cooked broccoli into a small ovenproof dish, cover with the crème fraiche mixture, sprinkle on the remaining cheese and grill for 3-4 minutes until golden.

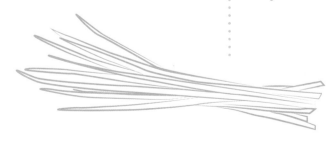

BABY CREAMY PEA PURÉE

YOU MINTED PEA HUMMUS WITH OATCAKES

Peas (both fresh and frozen) are a great source of vitamin C. This is one of the most important vitamins needed for a healthy immune system and can help protect both you and your baby from picking up colds and infections, which you can be more susceptible to once you start mixing in new mum and baby groups. They are a good source of fibre and protein. They also contain phytonutrients, which have antioxidant and anti-inflammatory benefits. Peas have a low GI and research has linked them to a lowered risk of type 2 diabetes.

Preparation time: 10 mins
Cooking time: 5 mins

TO PREPARE
One 200g frozen peas

FOR BABY
1 cube apple purée

2 tbsp peas

1 tsp Greek yogurt

FOR YOU
Makes 3 portions (the remainder can be kept in the fridge in an airtight container for up to 3 days)

The remaining peas

100g artichoke hearts (from a jar)

2 tsp (10 ml) ground cumin

2 tbsp (30 ml) lemon juice

2 tbsp (30 ml) olive oil

Small handful of mint leaves

Salt and pepper

Oatcakes to serve

Shop-bought hummus is fine, but this is far superior and well worth the tiny bit of effort involved. As you've made it fresh it will retain more of its vitamin content, which fades away in processed versions. And making your own means you can control the flavour (minty or spicy) and the texture (smooth or coarse). Serve on oatcakes which provide a slow release fibre and will keep your energy levels up.

Put the peas into a bowl and pour in enough boiling water to cover. Leave for 5 minutes and then drain and tip into a food processor and pulse to make a rough paste.

FOR BABY CREAMY PEA PURÉE
While the peas are soaking, remove a cube of puréed apple from the freezer and place in a bowl to defrost. Add 2 tbsp of the blended peas to the apple purée and blend using a handheld blender. Add 1 tsp of Greek yogurt and swirl through the purée.

FOR YOU MINTED PEA HUMMUS WITH OATCAKES
Drain the artichoke hearts and add to the peas in the food processor. Add the cumin, lemon juice, oil and mint leaves and pulse to make a rough paste. Transfer to a bowl and season to taste with the salt and pepper. Serve with the oatcakes.

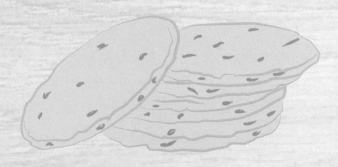

BABY CREAMY PUMPKIN & BANANA PURÉE
YOU SPICY PUMPKIN & BUTTER BEAN SOUP

Pumpkin provides plenty of nutrients that will boost your and your baby's immune system. Just a few slices of pumpkin will provide well over 100% of her daily needs for vitamin A, 20% of the daily value for vitamin C and 10% for vitamin E. It also provides B vitamins, potassium, iron and magnesium.

Preparation time: 2 mins for the squash/10 mins for the soup
Cooking time: 50-60 mins for the squash/10 mins for the soup

TO PREPARE
One 200g frozen peas

FOR BABY
2 tbsp (30ml) of the cooked pumpkin

1 cube frozen apple purée, thawed, or 1 tbsp (15ml) fresh apple purée

½ banana, roughly chopped

A little baby milk or plain Greek yogurt, sour cream or crème fraîche (optional)

FOR YOU
Serves 4

1 tbsp (15ml) olive oil

4 spring onions

1 tsp (5ml) garlic paste or 1 garlic clove, crushed

1 tsp (5ml) chilli paste

2 tsp (10ml) ras el hanout (Moroccan spice mix)

1 tsp (5ml) cumin seeds

400g canned chopped tomatoes

400g canned butter beans, drained

1 litre hot vegetable stock

The remaining cooked pumpkin

A handful of fresh coriander

Salt and ground black pepper

Fresh coriander leaves, to garnish

If you think a soup takes ages to cook, this super-fast one will soon change your mind. Everything is quick to cook and needs less than 10 minutes to simmer – perfect for when you come home from a busy morning out and about and don't want to give in to the lure of the cookie jar. This one is especially filling and tasty, and will keep you going until dinnertime.

Preheat the oven to 180°C (Gas 4). Use a heavy, sharp knife to cut the pumpkin in half, then scoop out the seeds (and set aside – see p.71) and discard the fibrous strings.

Put the pumpkin cut side down in a baking tray and add enough water to come 1cm up the sides of the pumpkin. Roast for 50–60 minutes, until tender. You can do this bit in the morning before you go out.

FOR BABY CREAMY PUMPKIN & BANANA PURÉE
Put the cooked pumpkin, apple and banana in a bowl. Use a fork to mash them together. Add a little baby milk or plain Greek yogurt, sour cream or crème fraîche if you want to achieve a slightly thinner consistency.

FOR YOU SPICY PUMPKIN & BUTTER BEAN SOUP
While the pumpkin is cooking, heat the oil in a large pan. Use scissors to snip the spring onions and add to the pan with the garlic, chilli, ras el hanout and cumin seeds. Cook for 3 minutes, then add the tomatoes, butter beans and stock and bring to the boil. Simmer for 7–8 minutes, then add the pumpkin pieces and most of the fresh coriander.

Blitz to form as smooth a soup as you like, using a hand-held blender or standard blender. Season with a pinch of salt and plenty of black pepper and serve with the reserved coriander leaves.

BABY CRUSHED BLUEBERRIES
YOU BLUEBERRY & SPINACH SMOOTHIE

Your baby will love sweet and delicious blueberries and they are regarded as one of nature's superfoods, packed with disease-fighting antioxidants and vitamins. They also benefit the brain and can help to improve memory. Despite their sweetness, blueberries have a low GI, meaning blood-sugar levels are kept even.

Preparation time: 5 mins
Cooking time: 0 mins

TO PREPARE
One punnet of blueberries

FOR BABY
2 tbsp (30ml) baby rice flakes

1 tbsp (15ml) plain Greek yogurt

1 tbsp (15ml) of the crushed blueberries

FOR YOU
Serves 1
¼ of a Galia melon

The remaining whole blueberries

2 handfuls of baby spinach leaves

200ml unsweetened almond milk

A sprinkle of sunflower seeds

Some mornings it will feel as though you have been up for hours but you're still running late, and it's tempting to run out of the house without eating. This super-fast, super-tasty and superfood-packed smoothie takes just 5 minutes to make, and is full of nutritional goodness that will really benefit your body. Use your regular milk if you don't have almond milk.

Put the blueberries in a bowl and gently crush them with the back of a spoon. Your baby will be able to manage the small bits of peel and pips, but they may give her runnier poo the first time she tries it. To prevent this, push the crushed blueberries through a fine-mesh sieve and serve your baby just the pulp.

FOR BABY CRUSHED BLUEBERRIES
Mix together all of the ingredients to form a smooth paste.

FOR YOU BLUEBERRY & SPINACH SMOOTHIE
Chop the melon, then put it in a blender with the berries, spinach and milk and whizz until smooth. Sprinkle on the sunflower seeds.

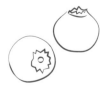

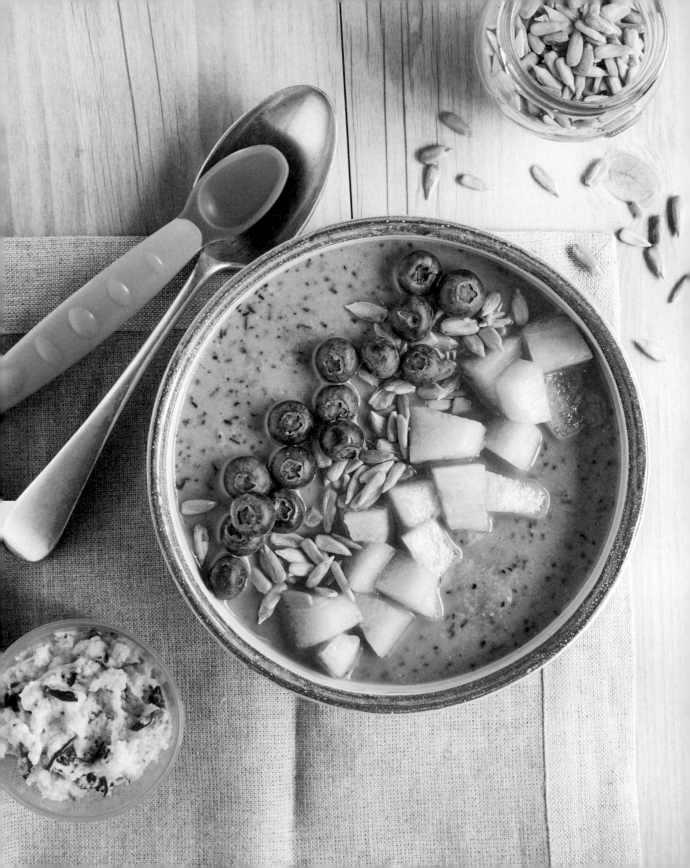

BABY CREAMY PRUNE PURÉE

YOU CHICKEN & RADISH SALAD WITH PRUNE DRESSING

Prunes are a great weaning food, providing iron, which your baby needs after six months as body stores start to deplete, and vitamin C, which helps the absorption of the iron into the body. As your baby starts solids, they may experience a little constipation (this is perfectly normal) and prunes are a good way to help alleviate the problem. You only need a small amount as a little goes a long way. For you, as well as beneficial iron and vitamin C, prunes contain two types of fibre – soluble and insoluble. The soluble fibre promotes a sense of satisfied fullness after a meal by slowing the rate at which food leaves the stomach, so prunes can also help prevent overeating and weight gain, while the insoluble fibre can help to lower cholesterol levels in the blood.

Preparation time: 10 mins
Cooking time: 8-10 mins

TO PREPARE
10 soft pitted prunes

FOR BABY
2 cubes of pear purée,
or 2 tbsp (30ml) fresh pear purée

2 tbsp (30ml) plain Greek yogurt

1 tbsp (15ml) of the puréed prunes

FOR YOU
Serves 1
1 cooked chicken breast

5 radishes

2 handfuls of baby spinach leaves

1 tbsp (15ml) hazelnuts

The remaining prune purée

1 tbsp (15ml) olive oil

1 tbsp (15ml) sherry vinegar

This is yet another perfect lunch if you're running on empty and need something fast. It's ready in minutes and the chicken is instantly satisfying (unlike carbohydrate foods such as white bread and pasta, which take time to process, meaning you can easily overeat). The peppery, crunchy radishes are a great contrast to the sticky sweet prunes.

Place the prunes in a small pan with 2 frozen cubes of pear purée and a splash of water (or the juice from the can or sachet) and bring to the boil. Reduce the heat and simmer for 8–10 minutes. Remove the pan from the heat and allow the mixture to cool. Transfer to a food processor or use a hand-held blender to whizz into a smooth paste.

FOR BABY CREAMY PRUNE PURÉE
Place the Greek yogurt into a bowl and swirl through the puréed prune mixture.

FOR YOU
CHICKEN & RADISH SALAD WITH PRUNE DRESSING
Shred the chicken and halve the radishes and place in a bowl with the spinach leaves and hazelnuts. Make the dressing by combining the prune mixture with the oil and vinegar and whisk together. Drizzle over the salad.

BABY CHEESY COURGETTE
YOU CHEESY CHICKPEA COURGETTES

It might surprise you to learn that courgettes are a lot more nutritious than they look! They contain good amounts of vitamin A, magnesium, folate, potassium, copper and phosphorus, and smaller but significant amounts of omega-3 fats and B vitamins. Although we're not counting calories it's worth noting that courgettes are particularly low in calories, containing only 15 calories each. Courgettes also play a role in promoting heart health. The nutrients magnesium and potassium help normalise blood pressure, while vitamins A and C stop the oxidation of bad cholesterol in the blood, reducing the risk of heart attacks. While vitamins A and C have an important role in looking after your heart as they are able to prevent the formation of plaques in the arteries (caused by the oxidation of bad cholesterol in the blood), this then lowers the risk of heart attacks.

Preparation time: 15 mins
Cooking time: 35 mins

TO PREPARE
2 courgettes

FOR BABY
A heaped tbsp (20ml) ricotta

2 cubes frozen butternut squash purée, thawed, or 2 tbsp (30ml) fresh butternut squash purée

1 hollowed-out courgette half

FOR YOU
Serves 1
1 fresh chilli

A handful of fresh herbs (mint, basil, parsley)

250g ricotta (minus the amount for your baby)

Grated rind of 1 lemon

2 tbsp (30ml) drained canned chickpeas

Salt and ground black pepper

The remaining hollowed-out courgette halves

1 tbsp (15ml) Parmesan cheese

This is a lovely light dish that you can liven up with a little chilli and whatever fresh herbs you have to hand – a mixture produces the most flavoursome and interesting result. The chickpeas add more protein and fibre to make the dish more substantial, but you could use any drained canned pulses or lentils.

Heat the oven to 200°C (Gas 6). Split the courgettes lengthways using a sharp knife. Use a teaspoon to scoop out the seeds from the middle of each courgette half, then place them in a large baking tray.

FOR BABY CHEESY COURGETTE
Mix together the ricotta and butternut squash purée. Don't worry if the cubes of purée (if using) are not fully defrosted – they will easily melt in the oven. Spoon the mixture into the hollowed-out courgette half and bake for about 35 minutes, until the courgette is very soft. Mash with a fork to form a thick, smooth purée.

FOR YOU CHEESY CHICKPEA COURGETTES
Deseed and finely chop the chilli and roughly tear the herbs. Mix together the ricotta, lemon zest, chilli, herbs and chickpeas, and season with salt and pepper.

Pile the stuffing into the three remaining courgette halves and sprinkle on the Parmesan.

Bake for 35 minutes, until the courgettes are tender and the topping is golden and crisp.

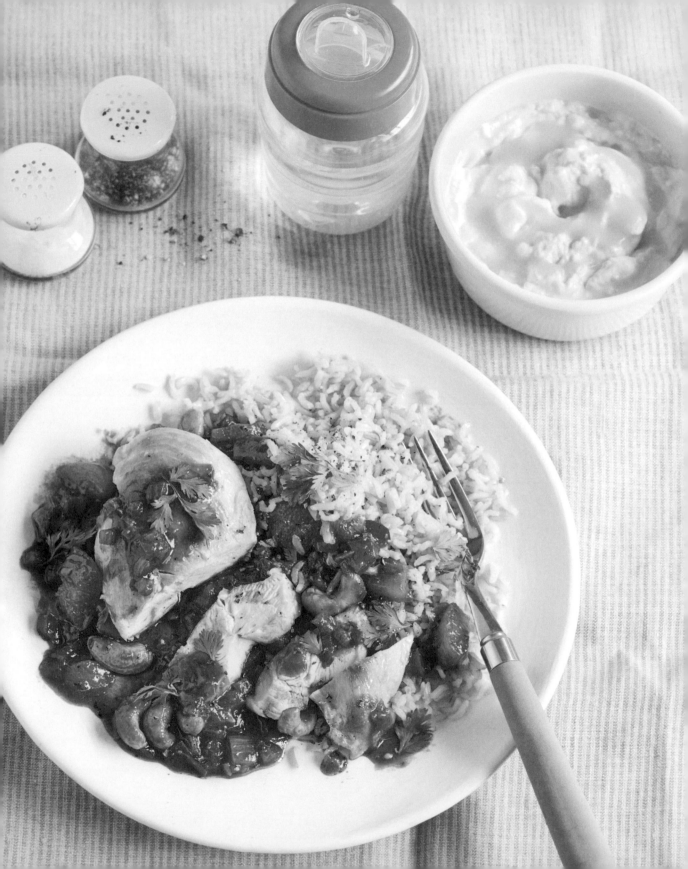

BABY APRICOT SWIRL
YOU SPICY APRICOT CHICKEN

Apricots are another low GI food that won't cause a spike in blood sugar. Instead, they release their energy slowly, which is much better for keeping hormone levels steady. Fresh apricots are not always in season or easy to get, so a can of apricot halves is a helpful substitute. Canned fruit still counts towards your five a day and only a few nutrients are lost during the canning process; vitamin C levels will be lower than in fresh apricots, but levels of other nutrients such as potassium, magnesium and folate remain unchanged. Choose apricots canned in juice rather than syrup.

Preparation time: 10 mins
Cooking time: 8-10 mins for the apricots/25 mins for apricot chicken

TO PREPARE
5 apricots (or a can of apricot halves)

2 cubes of frozen butternut squash purée

FOR BABY
1 tbsp (15ml) baby rice cereal

2 tbsp (30ml) plain Greek yogurt

2 tbsp (30ml) of the puréed apricots

FOR YOU
Serves 2
1 onion

1 celery stick

½ red pepper

The remaining half of the canned apricots or the remaining fresh apricot purée

1 tbsp (15ml) olive oil

2 skinless chicken breasts

100g uncooked brown basmati rice or 170g ready cooked brown basmati rice from a pouch

1 tsp (5ml) hot curry paste

2 tbsp (30ml) tomato purée

30g cashew nuts

100ml white wine or chicken stock

A handful of fresh coriander, to garnish

Here is a tasty dish to make for dinner for you and your partner; in fact, it's so simple even an inexperienced cook could give it a go. You can use dry brown basmati, or a ready steamed pouch for extra ease.

If using fresh apricots, take a sharp knife and make a slit around the stone. Prise open the fruit and remove the stone. Place all of the prepared fresh apricots or half of the canned apricots in a small pan with 2 frozen cubes of butternut squash purée and a splash of water (or the juice from the can) and bring to the boil. Reduce the heat and simmer for 8–10 minutes. Remove the pan from the heat and allow the mixture to cool. Transfer to a food processor and whizz into a smooth paste, or use a hand-held blender.

FOR BABY APRICOT SWIRL
Place the baby rice cereal and the Greek yogurt into a bowl, mix well and swirl through the puréed apricots..

FOR YOU SPICY APRICOT CHICKEN
Peel and finely chop the onion, finely chop the celery, deseed the pepper and cut into strips, and slice the tinned apricot halves, if using.

Heat the oil in a frying pan over a medium heat and add the chicken breasts. Cook for about 10 minutes on each side, making sure they are thoroughly cooked through. Remove from the pan and set aside.

Meanwhile, cook the rice according to the packet instructions. Add the onion, celery and pepper to the pan in which you cooked the chicken and cook for 10 minutes, until softened.

Stir in the curry paste, tomato purée, apricots, cashew nuts and wine or stock and bring to the boil. Reduce the heat and simmer for 5 minutes, until the sauce has reduced and become thicker.

Return the chicken breasts to the pan to heat through. Serve with the rice, garnished with fresh coriander leaves.

BABY CHEESY BAKED POTATO

YOU BAKED POTATO WITH SMOKED MACKEREL

The health benefits of potatoes are often overlooked, and many people hold the idea they are just full of bad carbs. Baked potatoes do have quite a high GI, which means if you were to eat the flesh it could potentially cause a blood-sugar spike. However, once the flesh cools down more of the fast-acting carbs turn to fibre and the GI lowers, so a healthier way to enjoy a baked potato is with a cold filling. Potatoes are also a good source of vitamin B$_6$, which is needed for the production of hormones in the brain that can keep you feeling calm and happy, and aid sleep. They also provide potassium, copper, vitamin C, manganese and B vitamins.

Preparation time: 10 mins
Cooking time: 30 or 50 mins

TO PREPARE
2 medium-sized baking potatoes

FOR BABY
½ baked potato

1 tbsp (15ml) crème fraîche, sour cream or plain Greek yogurt

1 tbsp (15ml) snipped chives

1 tbsp (15ml) grated cheese (such as mild Cheddar or mozzarella)

FOR YOU
Serves 1
6 mushrooms

1 spring onion

2 thin fillets of smoked mackerel

2 tbsp (30ml) crème fraîche, sour cream or plain Greek yogurt

Ground black pepper

The remaining baked potato halves

You are left with three potato halves, so make sure you choose medium-sized potatoes or, if you prefer, you can share one large potato with your baby and add extra salad to your plate. The smoked mackerel is a very rich source of omega-3 fats – needed to protect joints from inflammation and stiffness and improve mood.

Prick the potato five or six times all over with a knife tip or fork. You can either bake in the oven at 200ºC (Gas 6) for 50 minutes, or microwave on High for 10–12 minutes, turning it halfway through and checking for tenderness. If you prefer your potato to have a crispy skin and have the oven on already (it's not really worth turning it on just to crisp the skin), bake the microwaved potato at 200ºC (Gas 6) for 20 minutes.

FOR BABY CHEESY BAKED POTATO
Set the grill to high. Take one half of the baked potato, scoop out the flesh and place it in a bowl. Mix with the crème fraîche, sour cream or Greek yogurt, the snipped chives and the grated cheese. Place the mixture back into the skin and pop it under the grill for 1–2 minutes, until the cheese is melted and bubbling. Serve just the cheesy filling to your baby – not the skin.

FOR YOU BAKED POTATO WITH SMOKED MACKEREL
Slice the mushrooms and place on the baking sheet next to your baby's potato, and grill them at the same time as the potato. Transfer the mushrooms to a bowl.

Use scissors to cut the spring onion and add to the mushrooms. Flake off the mackerel flesh from the skin, and add to the bowl with the crème fraîche, sour cream or Greek yogurt. Season with black pepper, mix well to combine, then pile the topping on to the potato halves and serve.

Red peppers are a great source of carotenoids including beta-carotene, and roasting them in a little oil helps to release more of the carotenoids from the tough cell walls and makes it easier for the body to digest them. Beta-carotene is an important antioxidant needed by the immune system that protects cells in the body from damage caused by environmental toxins. Red peppers also provide vitamins C and E.

Preparation time: 10 mins
Cooking time: 15 mins

TO PREPARE
One red pepper

A drizzle of olive oil

FOR BABY
½ the roasted pepper flesh

2 cubes frozen apple purée, thawed, or 2 tbsp (30ml) fresh apple purée, plus extra if necessary

2 small slices from a pasteurised goat's cheese log

A drop of your baby's normal milk, if necessary

FOR YOU
Serves 1
40g pasteurised goat's cheese log

A pinch of dried oregano

1 large wholemeal pitta

A handful of rocket or baby spinach leaves

A handful of fresh herbs (basil, parsley)

The remaining roasted pepper

1 tbsp (15ml) black olives

A squeeze of lemon juice

The sweetness of the pepper contrasts nicely with the tanginess of the cheese in this dish. Add olives, herbs, lemon and rocket for a Mediterranean flavour.

Preheat the oven to 200°C (Gas 6). Cut the pepper in half lengthways and discard the seeds. Place the pepper open-side up on a baking tray and drizzle with a little olive oil. Bake for 15 minutes. Remove from the oven, then peel off the skin and roughly chop the flesh.

FOR BABY CHEESY PEPPER
Place the pepper into a food processor with the apple purée and cheese and whizz together to form a rough paste. If it seems too thick, thin it down with a little extra apple purée or a drop of your baby's normal milk.

FOR YOU RED PEPPER & GOAT'S CHEESE PITTA
Dice the goat's cheese and sprinkle it with the oregano.

Place the pitta in a toaster and toast until it puffs up. Remove from the toaster and carefully split along one side to open it up (take care as steam will escape from the inside).

Add the leaves and herbs, then the slices of roast pepper, the diced cheese and the olives. Squeeze over a little lemon juice and close up.

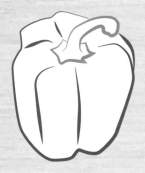

BABY SPINACH WITH GREEN LENTILS
YOU SPICY SPINACH & LENTIL SOUP

Preparation time: 15 mins
Cooking time: 7-8 mins

TO PREPARE
1 bag of baby spinach leaves

FOR BABY
1/3 of the cooked spinach

1 cube frozen apple purée , thawed,
or 1 tbsp (15ml) fresh apple purée

1 cube frozen pear purée, thawed,
or 1 tbsp (15ml) fresh pear purée

1 tbsp (15ml) cooked green lentils
(from a pouch or can)

1 tbsp (15ml) plain Greek yogurt,
sour cream or crème fraîche

FOR YOU
Serves 2

1 tbsp (15ml) olive oil

1 tsp (5ml) garlic paste
or 1 garlic clove, crushed

1 tsp (5ml) lemongrass paste
(or a squeeze of lemon juice added at the end)

A pinch of chilli flakes

1 tsp (5ml) cumin seeds

1 tsp (5ml) paprika

2 spring onions

200g cooked green lentils (from a pouch or can)

800ml vegetable or chicken stock

1 tbsp (15ml) tomato purée

Salt and ground black pepper

2 tomatoes

The remaining spinach

Plain Greek yogurt, sour cream
or crème fraîche, to serve

One of the most important nutritional aspects of spinach is its high iron content. Your baby needs a regular source of iron in his diet now because the stores he was born with will be starting to decline. You may also be low in iron, particularly if you had a traumatic birth or you lost a lot of blood. A poor intake of iron can leave you feeling fatigued and easily out of breath and eventually result in anaemia.

Spinach is also an excellent source of vitamins K, A, and C, and folate, as well as being a good source of manganese, magnesium and B vitamins. Vitamin K is important for maintaining bone health and it is difficult to find a vegetable richer in it than spinach.

The addition of lentils adds protein and fibre to make this delicious soup more satisfying. Lentils release their energy slowly, helping you to feel energised all afternoon, and will help prevent the mid-afternoon craving for something sweet. Like the spinach, lentils are also a good source of iron, so this soup will give your body a real power shot and top up any depleted stores.

Bring 2.5cm water in a pan to the boil. Place the spinach leaves in a steamer basket or sieve, position over the water, cover tightly with a lid or an upturned plate and allow to steam for 2–3 minutes.

Drain and squeeze the leaves to remove any excess water.

FOR BABY SPINACH WITH GREEN LENTILS
Place the spinach in a food processor with the purées and whizz together. Add the cooked green lentils and pulse to form a coarse paste. Transfer to a bowl and swirl through the Greek yogurt, sour cream or crème fraîche.

FOR YOU SPICY SPINACH & LENTIL SOUP
Heat the oil in a pan and add the garlic paste, lemongrass paste (if using), chilli flakes, cumin seeds and paprika and cook for 1 minute.

Using scissors, cut the spring onions, add them to the pan and cook for another minute. Add the lentils, stock and tomato purée and bring to the boil. Season with a pinch of salt and plenty of black pepper.

Dice the tomatoes and add to the spinach. Stir to combine, then simmer for 5 minutes.

Serve with a dollop of yogurt and a squeeze of lemon juice (if using).

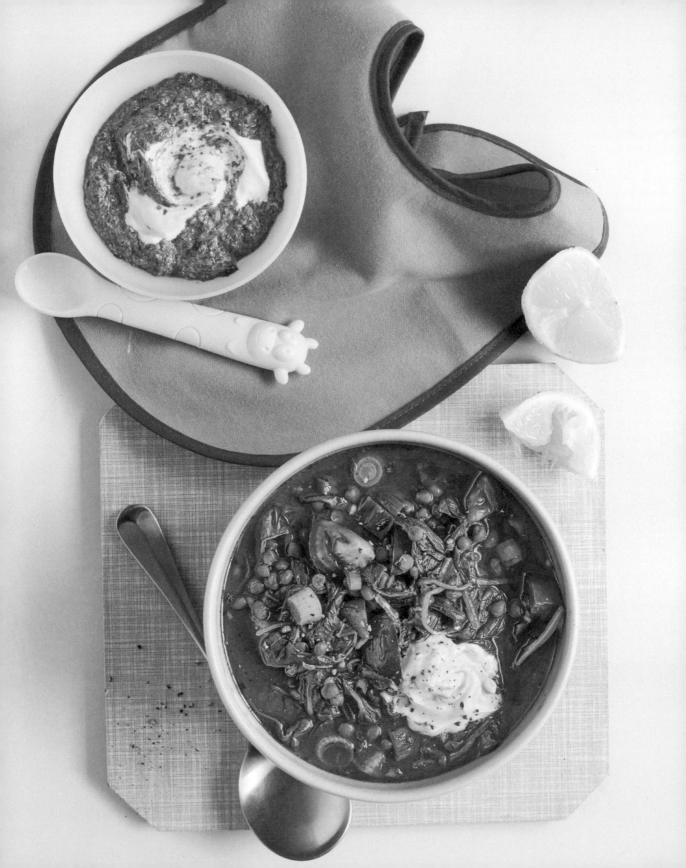

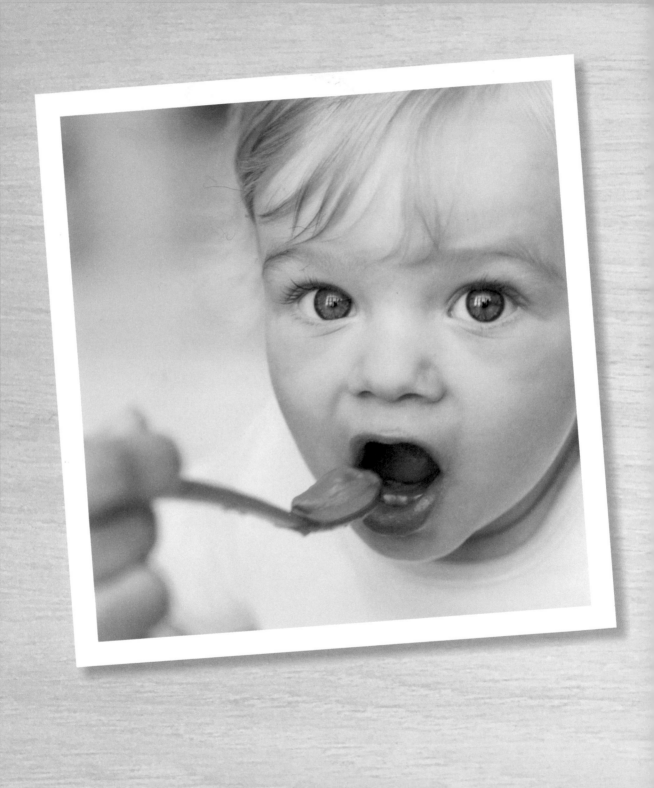

BABY CARROT DHAL
YOU CARROT & GINGER PÂTÉ

This is a lovely vibrant pâté that is bursting with flavour. The peanut butter gives it a mild flavour (and some texture, if you use the crunchy type), while the tahini has a more pungent flavour and smooth consistency; both work equally well.

Preparation time: 15 mins
Cooking time: 5 mins

TO PREPARE
2 carrots or a bag of spiralised carrot

FOR BABY
1 cube frozen butternut squash purée, thawed, or 1 tbsp/15ml fresh butternut squash purée

1 cube frozen apple purée, thawed, or 1 tbsp/15ml fresh apple purée

2 tbsp (30ml) of the carrot purée

A pinch of mild curry powder

A pinch of ground cumin

1 tbsp (15ml) cooked chickpeas (from a pouch or can)

FOR YOU
Serves 1
Carrot and ginger pate

The remaining carrot purée

1 tsp (5ml) ginger paste

2 tbsp (30ml) drained canned chickpeas

1 tbsp (15ml) smooth or crunchy peanut butter or tahini

Juice of ½ lemon

1 tbsp (15ml) olive oil

A handful of coriander leaves

Salt and ground black pepper

Wholegrain toast, to serve

Peel the carrots and spiralise. Spiralising the carrot will allow them to cook much more quickly. Place in a saucepan of boiling water and simmer until tender for 2-3 minutes. Drain and place in a food processor and blend into a purée.

Put all of the ingredients in a pan (re-use the pan in which you cooked the carrots if you are making this straight afterwards). Gently heat through, then mash with a fork. If you prefer a really smooth consistency, whizz the mixture in a blender.

FOR BABY CARROT DHAL
While the carrots are cooking defrost a cube each of butternut squash and apple. Transfer 2 tbsp of puréed carrot into a bowl and mix with the other purées. Add a pinch of mild curry powder and a pinch of ground cumin. Stir in a tbsp of cooked chickpeas (from a pouch or can). Transfer back to the saucepan and gently heat though and then mash gently with a fork.

FOR YOU CARROT & GINGER PÂTÉ
Add all the ingredients to the carrots already in the food processor and whizz together to make a coarse paste. Transfer to a bowl and season with a pinch of salt and plenty of black pepper and serve on wholegrain toast.

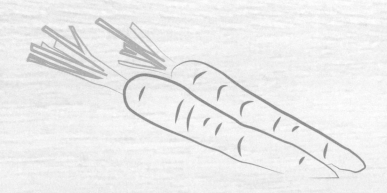

BABY PARSNIP & APPLE PURÉE
YOU CRAB CAKES

Parsnips have a mild, sweet taste but are not high in natural sugars; in fact they contain high amounts of soluble fibre, which keeps blood-sugar levels balanced, fills you up and prevent the release of ghrelin, which is a 'hunger' hormone. This can significantly reduce your likelihood of snacking between meals. Parsnips also contain high levels of potassium, manganese, magnesium, phosphorous, zinc, and iron, as well as B vitamins and vitamins C, E, and K.

Preparation time: 25 mins
Cooking time: 15-20 mins

TO PREPARE
2 large parsnips

1tsp (15ml) crème fraîche

200g (small can) butter beans

FOR BABY

2 tbsp (30ml) of the parsnip mixture

2 cubes frozen apple purée, thawed, or 2 tbsp (30ml) fresh apple purée

FOR YOU
Makes 4
2 spring onions

A handful of fresh coriander

The remaining parsnip mixture

250g white crabmeat

1 tbsp (15ml) hot horseradish sauce

2 eggs

1 tbsp (15ml) water

Plain flour, for dusting

8 tbsp (120ml) wholemeal breadcrumbs

2 tbsp (30ml) olive oil

Fresh green salad, to serve

The parsnip and butterbean mixture makes a nutritious base for these tasty crab cakes – just chill it in the fridge before you combine the ingredients or they won't bind together. As well as upping the protein content, the crabmeat is also a great source of iodine, zinc and selenium.

Peel and roughly chop the parsnips and place in a pan of boiling water. Simmer for 10 minutes, until tender. Drain. Alternatively, place in a suitable dish and microwave the chopped parsnip with a little water, covered, on High for about 8 minutes, checking and stirring them halfway through the cooking time.

Transfer the soft parsnips to a food processor with 1 tbsp (15ml) crème fraîche. Drain a small can (about 200g) of butter beans and add to the processor, then whizz together to make a coarse paste.

FOR BABY PARSNIP & APPLE PURÉE
Put the parsnip mixture and apple purée into a small pan and gently heat.

FOR YOU CRAB CAKES
Use scissors to chop the spring onions, then roughly tear the coriander leaves. Add to the bowl of chilled parsnip mixture, along with the crabmeat and horseradish. Stir to combine.

Beat one of the eggs, then add it to the bowl and mix until everything is well combined. Using damp hands, form the mixture into a rough 'cake', then divide it into quarters and form each wedge into a patty. The mixture should already be cold from the fridge, but if it doesn't handle well, place it in the fridge for 5 minutes more to firm up a little.

When you are ready to cook, preheat the oven to 180°C (Gas 4). Beat the remaining egg in a small bowl with the water to make an egg wash. Place some plain flour and the breadcrumbs in two separate shallow dishes.

Dust each fishcake with flour, then dip in the beaten egg and finally the breadcrumbs, making sure they are evenly coated. Shake gently to remove any excess breadcrumbs.

Heat the olive oil in a frying pan and fry the fishcakes for 2–3 minutes on each side, or until crisp and golden-brown all over.

Transfer to a baking tray and bake in the oven for 5–10 minutes, or until piping hot all the way through. Serve with a fresh green salad.

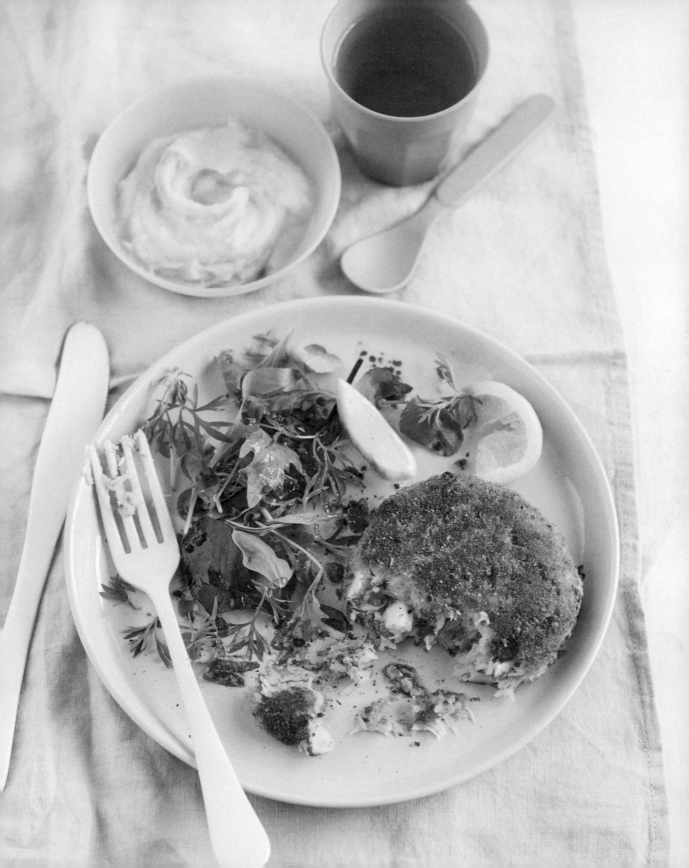

BABY CAULIFLOWER CHEESE
YOU 'PIMPED' CAULIFLOWER CHEESE

Cauliflower is an excellent source of vitamin C, and a very good source of manganese: two of the key antioxidant nutrients the body needs to stay healthy. As your baby grows and develops, cells are replicating continuously and these antioxidant nutrients protect the cells from damage and ensure healthy growth.

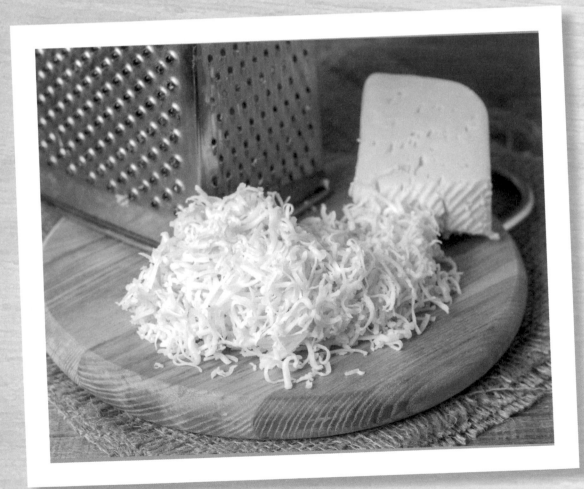

Preparation time: 25 mins
Cooking time: 55 mins

TO PREPARE
1 head of cauliflower

FOR BABY
¼ of the cooked cauliflower

**2 cubes frozen pear purée, thawed,
or 2 tbsp (30ml) fresh pear purée**

A pat of butter

1 tbsp (15ml) crème fraîche

1 tbsp (15ml) ricotta

**A handful of grated mild cheese,
such as Cheddar or Edam**

FOR YOU
Serves 2
1 leek

A pat of butter

100g pancetta

250ml milk

1 tbsp (15ml) butter

1 tbsp (15ml) plain flour

**1 tsp (5ml) garlic paste
or 1 garlic clove, crushed**

A pinch of ground black pepper

A pinch of freshly grated nutmeg

100g mature Cheddar cheese, grated

The remaining cooked cauliflower

2 large handfuls of spinach leaves

1 tbsp (15ml) Parmesan cheese

1 slice of wholemeal bread

50g flaked almonds

A handful of fresh thyme leaves

6 cherry tomatoes

Save the rest of the cauliflower to make this comforting supper – just what you need after a busy day. It might be comfort food but the addition of extra veg and nuts make it a balanced and nutritious meal.

Trim the outer leaves from the cauliflower and then cut off even-sized florets. Place in a pan of boiling water and simmer for 12–15 minutes, until tender. Drain off any excess water.

FOR BABY CAULIFLOWER CHEESE
Set the grill to high. Place a quarter of the cauliflower florets into a food processor with the pear purée. Add the butter, crème fraîche and ricotta and whizz together until smooth.

Transfer the mixture into a heatproof dish and sprinkle with a handful of grated cheese. Place under the preheated grill for a minute or so, until golden.

FOR YOU 'PIMPED' CAULIFLOWER CHEESE
While the cauliflower is cooking preheat the oven to 180°C (Gas 4). Finely slice the leek, then melt the butter in a frying pan over a low heat. Sweat the leeks in the butter for about 5 minutes, stirring occasionally, until softened.

While the leeks cook, chop the pancetta (if necessary) into small pieces and add to the frying pan with the sweated-down leeks. Turn up the heat to high and stir constantly for 8–10 minutes, until the leeks have reduced and the pancetta is beginning to go crispy.

Heat up the milk in a pan or microwave so that it is just hot but not boiling. Melt the 1 tbsp (15ml) butter in a large pan, then add the flour and the garlic and cook it on a high heat for about 1 minute, until it clumps together to form a soft, shiny ball. Add the milk, little by little, stirring after each addition continuously with a wooden spoon or a whisk to ensure no lumps form. Once all the milk has been added, season with black pepper and nutmeg.

Turn down the heat to medium and stir in the grated cheese, reserving a handful for the topping. Stir until all the cheese has melted. Remove from the heat.

Place the cauliflower and spinach leaves in an ovenproof dish. Scatter over the leeks and pancetta, then pour over the cheese sauce.

Place the Parmesan, bread, almonds and thyme leaves in a food processor, whizz together to form breadcrumbs, then scatter over the cauliflower cheese. Halve the cherry tomatoes and dot them over the top. Sprinkle over the remaining grated Cheddar and bake in the oven for 20–25 minutes, until golden.

BABY MANGO PORRIDGE

YOU TUNA WITH MANGO & AVOCADO SALSA

Despite tasting sweet, mangoes have a low GI and studies have shown that people who eat mangoes have a lower risk of developing diabetes. Mangoes are a rich source of vitamin C and beta-carotene, and provide fibre that can lower cholesterol levels and promote healthy bacteria in the gut.

Preparation time: 10 mins
Cooking time: 12 mins

TO PREPARE
1 mango

FOR BABY
½ of the mango cubes

150ml milk

A pinch of ground mixed spice

3 tbsp (45ml) fine porridge oats

FOR YOU
Serves 2
1 small avocado

1 small red onion

1 red chilli

A handful of fresh coriander leaves

A handful of fresh mint leaves

The remaining mango cubes

Juice of 1 lime

2 tbsp (30ml) olive oil, plus extra for drizzling

2 tuna steaks

Salt and ground black pepper

Sugar snap peas, to serve

Use the remaining mango to make this spicy salsa. It will go well with white fish or chicken, but I have chosen fresh tuna as it is such a nutritious fish, providing omega-3 fats, protein and other many other good things; think of this dish as a little beauty aid, since it gives you minerals including selenium, iodine and zinc, which are needed for healthy hair and nails. The avocado is a great source of vitamin E, which helps to keep skin looking smooth.

Slice the mango lengthways across one side of the stone. Remove the stone and then score the flesh of each half lengthways and across, to form a grid pattern. Place both thumbs on the skin and push outwards to make a mango 'hedgehog'. Run your knife close to the skin to cut away the little cubes of mango into a bowl positioned underneath (this will catch the juice too, which would run off a chopping board).

FOR BABY MANGO PORRIDGE
Place the mango cubes into a small pan with a splash of the milk and the mixed spice and cook for 2–3 minutes, until the mango softens. Add the fine porridge oats to the pan with the remaining milk, stir well, then bring to the boil and simmer for 3 minutes.

FOR YOU TUNA WITH MANGO & AVOCADO SALSA
Cut the avocado in half, remove and discard the stone, then peel away the skin. Dice the avocado flesh. Peel and finely dice the onion. Deseed (if you like) the chilli, then finely dice it. Roughly chop the herbs.

Place all of the prepared ingredients into a bowl and add the mango, lime juice and olive oil. Mix to combine. Chill in the fridge until ready to serve.

Drizzle each tuna steak with a little olive oil and rub all over the fish, then season well with salt and pepper. Place a ridged griddle pan over a high heat and add the tuna steaks. Cook for 3 minutes, then turn over and cook for 3 minutes on the other side, until charred and just cooked through.

Serve the tuna steaks with some sugar snap peas and the salsa on the side.

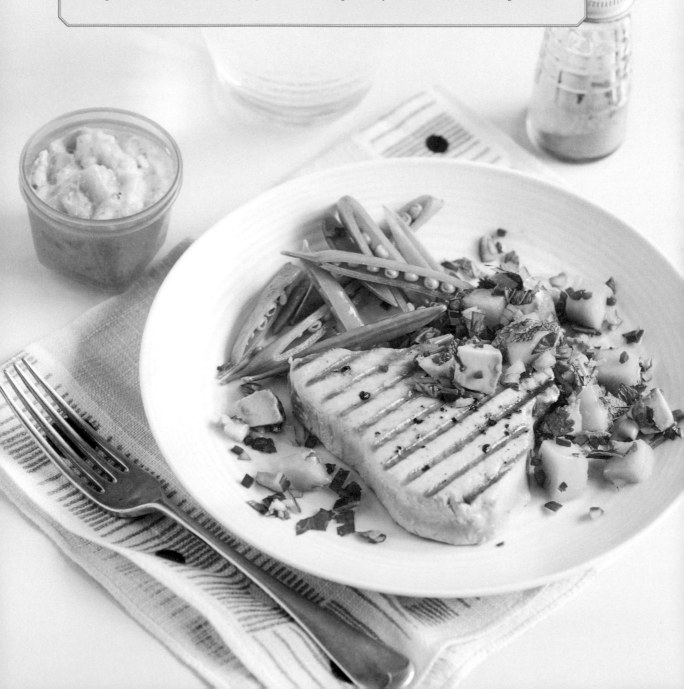

THAWING FROZEN PURÉES

Freezing purées in ice-cube trays is an extremely convenient and easy way to ensure your baby receives a range of different foods in one day, without you having to spend hours in the kitchen. They take very little time to defrost: simply put them in a bowl when you start cooking the other ingredients for whatever combination purée you are making (if applicable), and leave them at room temperature. It doesn't matter if they aren't completely defrosted when you add them to other ingredients if those are hot anyway. Allow a little longer if they will be mixed with cold ingredients.

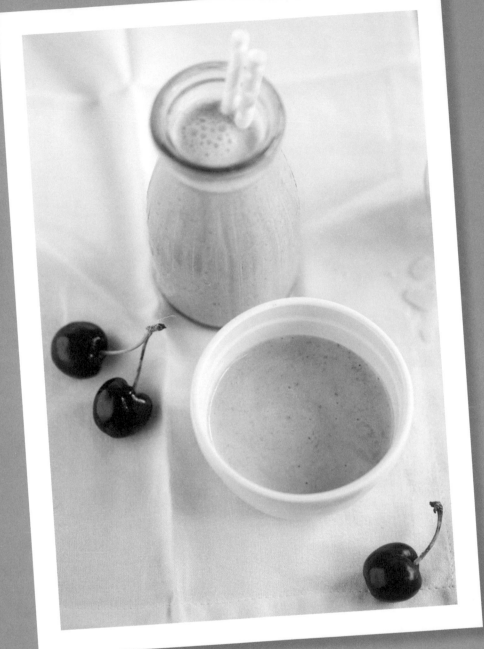

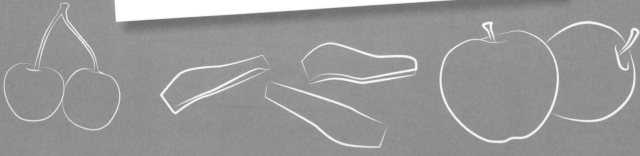

STAGE 2
BREAKFASTS

Up until now you may have been skipping breakfast or grabbing a few biscuits as you struggle through chaotic mornings. But now that your baby is ready to start having a regular breakfast, this is your opportunity to start a new healthy habit and share breakfast together. Some mornings you won't have much time or appetite, especially if you have been up all night trying to soothe your teething or unsettled little one. On those occasions a slice of wholemeal toast with peanut butter and a cup of tea is fine. But when you can, you want what you eat for breakfast to be more than just fuel. Go for foods that can keep you feeling energised, that are satisfying enough not to leave you feeling hungry all morning, and that provide nourishment for your body. These are the foods that you would select for your baby, so you should eat them too.

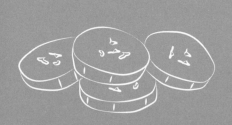
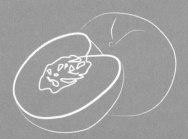

BABY PEACHES WITH YOGURT & OATMEAL

YOU HOLIDAY BREAKFAST

Peaches are an excellent source of beta-carotene, as well as being a good source of vitamin C, copper, dietary fibre and potassium. Peaches have been associated with a reduced risk of obesity related illnesses. Researchers attribute the health benefits of peaches to their content of four important phenolic substances which work together to keep the body healthy.

Preparation time 10 mins
Cooking time 6-8 mins

TO PREPARE
1 tsp (5ml) olive oil

1 tbsp (15ml) fresh lime juice

1 tsp (5ml) ground cinnamon

2 peaches

FOR BABY
150ml milk

3 tbsp (45ml) fine oatmeal

A pinch of cinnamon

2 of the grilled peach halves

1 tbsp (15ml) plain Greek yogurt

FOR YOU
Serves 1

The remaining 2 grilled peach halves

200g plain Greek yogurt

50g raspberries

1 tbsp (15ml) roughly chopped hazelnuts

A handful of fresh mint leaves, torn

I call this a 'holiday breakfast' as it will instantly lift your spirits and improve your mood. It provides a good balance of protein, carbohydrates, healthy fats and fibre as well as nourishing vitamins and minerals.

Preheat the grill to high. In a small bowl, combine the olive oil, lime juice, and cinnamon and whisk to blend. Set aside.

Split the peaches and remove the stones. Lightly brush the peaches with the marinade. Place under the hot grill, turning once and basting once or twice with the remaining marinade, until tender and golden – about 3–5 minutes on each side.

FOR BABY PEACHES WITH YOGURT & OATMEAL
Pour the milk into a small pan and add the fine oatmeal and cinnamon. Bring to the boil and simmer for 3 minutes. Roughly chop the peach and stir into the porridge. Transfer to a bowl and stir in the Greek yogurt.

FOR YOU HOLIDAY BREAKFAST
Serve the grilled peaches with the yogurt, scattered with the raspberries, hazelnuts and mint.

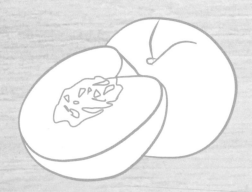

BABY PLUM AMARANTH
YOU YOGURT WITH PLUM COMPOTE

Plums are a very good source of vitamin C. They are also a good source of vitamin K, copper, dietary fibre and potassium. Their sweetness can vary according to variety and how ripe they are, so test a raw one first to ensure that it is naturally sweet enough to be palatable for your baby without the need for any additional sweetener once it has been cooked. Like quinoa, amaranth is an ancient grain, naturally gluten free, and rich in protein, fibre and minerals including magnesium, iron and selenium.

Preparation time 2 mins
Cooking time 20 mins

TO PREPARE
400g plums

Zest and juice of 1 orange

Zest and juice of 1 lemon

1 tsp (5ml) ginger paste

FOR BABY
150ml boiling water

3 tbsp (45ml) amaranth (available from health-food stores or some major supermarkets)

1 tbsp (15ml) plum compote

FOR YOU
Serves 1
2 tbsp (30ml) plum compote

200g plain Greek yogurt

Aim to make the plum compote the day before, so it's there to use when you are feeling hungry and exhausted and need a healthy pick-me-up.

Preheat the oven to 180°C (Gas 4). Slice the plums and remove the stones, then roughly chop the flesh. Put the plums, orange and lemon zest and juice, and the ginger in an ovenproof dish. Bake, uncovered, for 20 minutes.

Allow to cool, then transfer to an airtight container. This compote will keep in the fridge for 1–2 days.

FOR BABY PLUM AMARANTH
Pour the boiling water into a small pan and add the amaranth. Bring back to the boil and stir well, then cover the pan and reduce the heat. Allow to simmer for 20 minutes, stirring occasionally. When ready, the amaranth will be translucent, thick and sticky. Stir in the plum compote.

FOR YOU YOGURT WITH PLUM COMPOTE
Simply swirl the plum compote through the Greek yogurt and serve.

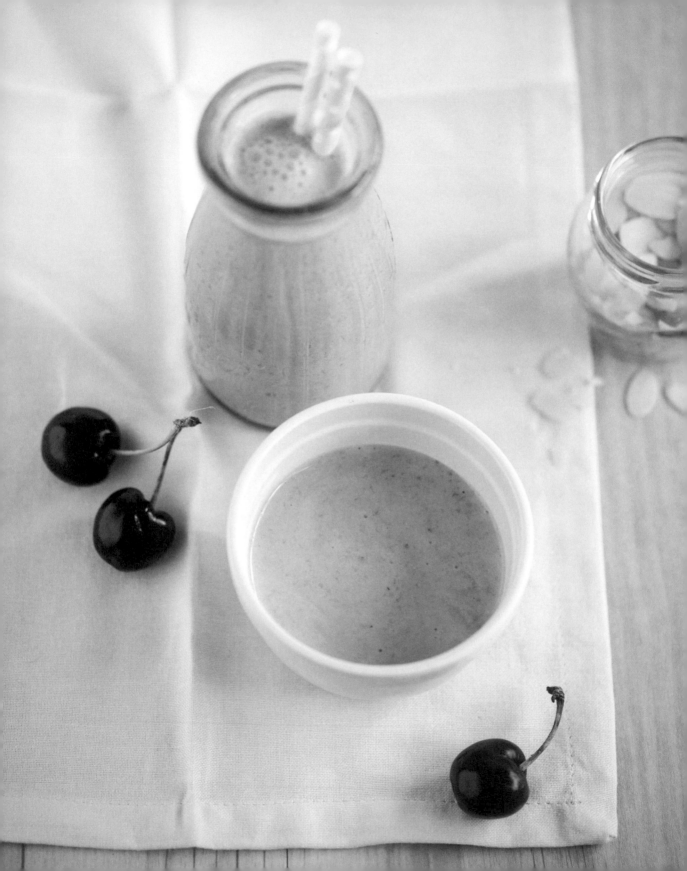

BABY CHERRY FROMAGE FRAIS
YOU CHERRY & GREEN TEA SMOOTHIE

Cherries are one of the few natural sources of melatonin, a hormone responsible for the regulation of the body's internal clock and sleep cycle. They are also high in substances known as anthocyanins, and it is the combination of these substances that are thought to promote sleep and help you overcome insomnia. Even when you are dog tired and sleep deprived you can suffer from insomnia when you have a new baby. Getting a good night's sleep is so important as being tired isn't just about feeling grumpy; while a restful night can lead to a more productive day, inadequate sleep is linked to sugar cravings, weight gain and high blood pressure.

Preparation time: 15 mins
Cooking time: 0 mins

TO PREPARE
110g of cherries

FOR BABY
1 tbsp (15ml) of the cherry purée
50g plain fromage fraîs

FOR YOU
Serves 1
1 green tea bag
2 tbsp (30ml) cherry purée
2 tbsp (30ml) Greek yogurt
1 tbsp (15ml) almonds
1 tbsp (15ml) flaxseed

This smoothie is great if you have a little more time; the cherries will take some time to stone, but it's worth the effort since this drink will give you a real injection of antioxidants from the green tea as well as the fruit. The almonds, flaxseed and yogurt add protein to help you feel full until lunchtime.

Carefully cut in half 100g cherries and remove the stones. Place the flesh in a blender and whizz together. Take care, as the juice stains! This purée will keep for a couple of days in a covered container in the fridge.

FOR BABY CHERRY FROMAGE FRAIS
Blend together the cherry purée and plain fromage fraîs.

FOR YOU CHERRY & GREEN TEA SMOOTHIE
Steep the green tea in a mug of boiling water for 3–4 minutes. Remove the teabag and pour the tea into the blender with the cherries. Add the Greek yogurt, almonds and flaxseed and blend together until smooth. Add a couple of ice cubes if you prefer your smoothie to be ice cold.

Whizz everything together. You could double up the quantity, although the benefits from the green tea will diminish over time so it is probably best made fresh.

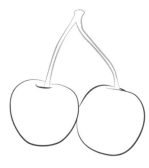

BABY MELON DIPPERS

YOU MELON, RASPBERRY & SPINACH SMOOTHIE

Melon is an excellent source of beta-carotene and vitamin C. It is also a very good source of potassium and a good source of dietary fibre, B vitamins, magnesium, copper, and vitamin K. Melon contains high amounts of substances which have anti-inflammatory properties. This reduces the level of background inflammation in the body and so reduces the risk of developing metabolic syndrome and diabetes.

Preparation time: 5 mins
Cooking time: 0 mins

TO PREPARE
A large wedge of honeydew melon

FOR BABY
2–3 of the melon slices

A small pot of soft white cheese

FOR YOU
Serves 1
The remaining melon slices

50g raspberries

2 handfuls of baby leaf spinach

1 tsp (5ml) chia seeds

Juice of 1 lime

200ml coconut water

This is the smoothie to choose when you have limited time and a busy morning ahead. The fibre in the melon means that energy is slowly released into your body, so you feel both energised and calm, which is ideal when dealing with the unpredictable and stressful situations that can arise when looking after a baby.

Cut a large wedge of Honeydew melon. Remove the seeds, then slice the flesh away from the skin and cut it into thick slices.

FOR BABY MELON DIPPERS
Encourage your baby to pick up the melon slices and dip them into a small pot of soft white cheese. She will love the chance to feed herself and enjoy dipping the melon into whatever is around – you've been warned!

FOR YOU MELON, RASPBERRY & SPINACH SMOOTHIE
Place all of the ingredients in a food processor and whizz together.

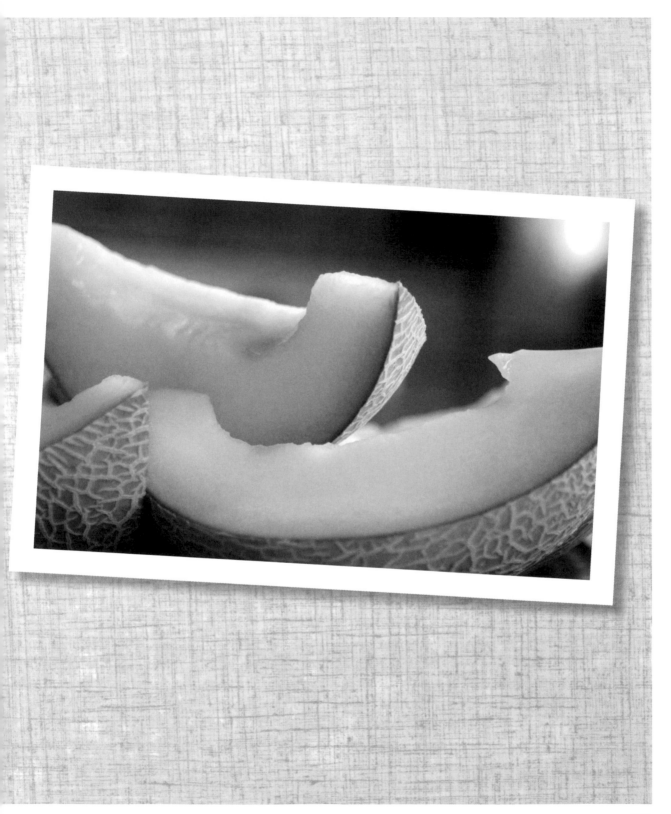

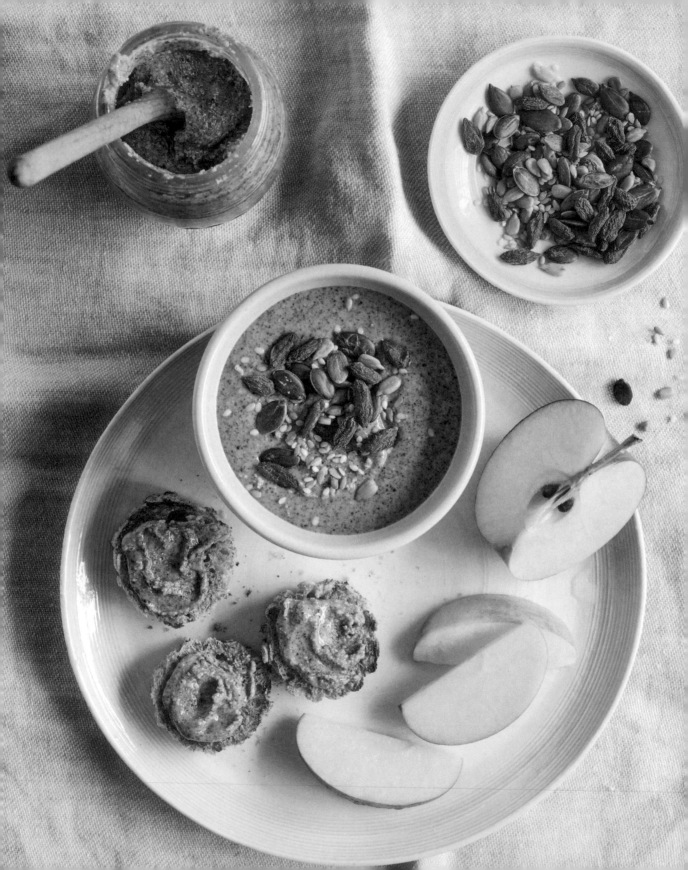

BABY ALMOND BUTTER ON TOAST
YOU ALMOND BUTTER WITH SEEDS, GOJI BERRIES & APPLE

Don't be afraid to introduce nut butters into your baby's diet. The recommendation to avoid nuts before the age of five years only applies to whole nuts and is due to the risk of choking. New advice is to introduce potentially allergenic foods earlier during weaning rather than later, as this lowers the chance of an initial allergic reaction. Once introduced, continue to offer these foods on a regular basis so the body becomes used to them. Almonds are extremely nutritious, containing protein, healthy fat and fibre. They are a very good source of vitamin E, manganese, biotin and copper and provide good amounts of magnesium, molybdenum, riboflavin and phosphorus.

Preparation time: 5 mins
Cooking time: 10 mins

TO PREPARE
300g skin-on almonds

FOR BABY
Some of the almond butter
1 slice toast

FOR YOU
Serves 1
2 tbsp (30ml) almond butter
2 tsp (10ml) mixed seeds
2 tsp (10ml) goji berries
1 apple

This is a protein-packed breakfast that is good for those mornings when you want to avoid the temptations of the indulgent coffees and sticky cakes at the local cafe. More protein in the morning will keep you feeling satisfied and prevent hunger pangs later.

Heat the oven to 190°C (Gas 5). Place 300g skin-on almonds on a baking sheet and bake in the oven for 10 minutes. This gives the almonds a toasted flavour and also helps to release their oils, which makes it easier to turn them into a butter.

Remove from the oven and place the warm almonds in a food processor. Process for 1–2 minutes, until finely ground, then stop and scrape down the sides. Blitz again for another few minutes, until smooth and creamy, stopping frequently so that the blender doesn't overheat. It is likely that the butter will not be as smooth as commercial almond butter, unless you have a very powerful blender, but the results will still be good and you will know it contains only almonds.

Transfer to a clean container or sterilised jars and store in the refrigerator for up to four weeks.

FOR BABY ALMOND BUTTER ON TOAST
Spread the almond butter on a slice of toast and cut into fingers.

FOR YOU
ALMOND BUTTER WITH SEEDS, GOJI BERRIES & APPLE
Put the almond butter in a dish and sprinkle with the mixed seeds and goji berries. Cut the apple into wedges and dip these in the mixture.

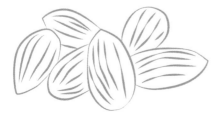

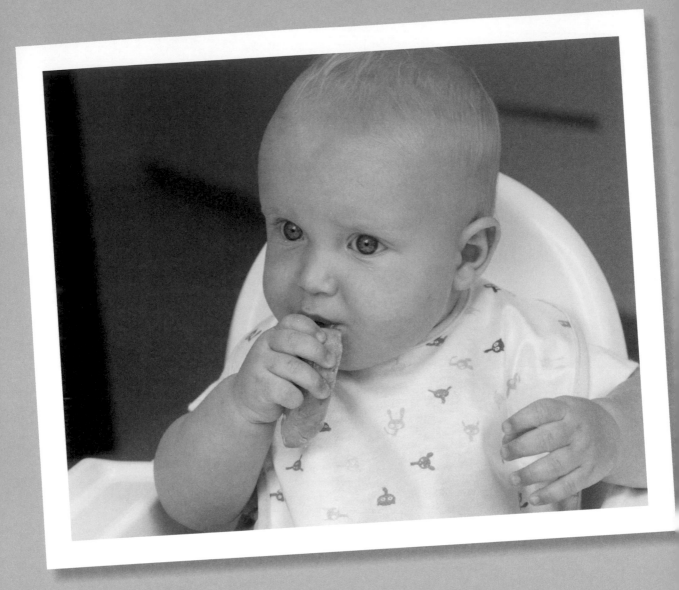

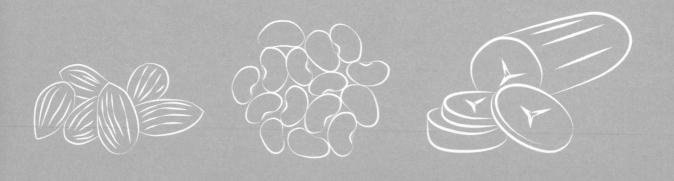

STAGE 2
SHARED LUNCHES

If you've had a busy morning it can be tempting to open a ready-made pouch of something for your baby and grab a few biscuits for yourself, so these lunches are not only tasty and nutritious they are really quick to make. Just take one shared ingredient and enjoy together.

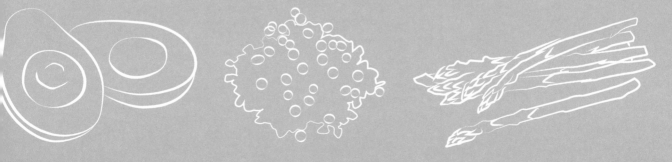

BABY CHEESY ASPARAGUS & APPLE PURÉE WITH ASPARAGUS WANDS

YOU ASPARAGUS & ALMOND SALAD

Asparagus is a very good source of fibre, folate, vitamins A, C, E and K, as well as chromium – a trace mineral with a vital role in balancing blood sugars. Folate is an important nutrient for helping ward off depression. It helps to balance hormones in the body and promotes the production of the feel-good hormones such as serotonin, which regulate mood, appetite and sleep.

Preparation time: 5 mins
Cooking time: 3-4 mins

TO PREPARE
100g asparagus spears

FOR BABY
⅓ of the cooked asparagus spears

2 cubes frozen apple purée, thawed, or 2 tbsp (30ml) fresh apple purée

1 tbsp (15ml) ricotta

FOR YOU
Serves 1
The remaining cooked asparagus spears

2 tbsp (30ml) flaked almonds

A squeeze of lemon juice

1 tbsp (15ml) grated cheese, such as Manchego

Cooked shredded chicken (optional)

This is a lovely lunch when you just fancy something light and easy. Socialising can be a big part of being a new parent and that can often mean plenty of tea and biscuits on offer. This salad is just enough to take the edge of your appetite so you won't feel tempted to over-indulge on unhealthy choices later in the day.

Remove the woody ends from the asparagus spears and add them to a pan of boiling water. Cook for 3–4 minutes, until tender. Drain and place in a bowl with a pat of butter, then gently toss so the melted butter coats the spears.

FOR BABY
CHEESY ASPARAGUS & APPLE PURÉE
WITH ASPARAGUS WANDS
Set aside a couple of asparagus spears for your baby to hold and gnaw upon while you are feeding her, then mash together the remaining spears with the apple purée and ricotta.

FOR YOU ASPARAGUS & ALMOND SALAD
Put the buttery asparagus on a plate and top with the almonds, lemon juice and cheese. Add some cooked shredded chicken if you want something more substantial.

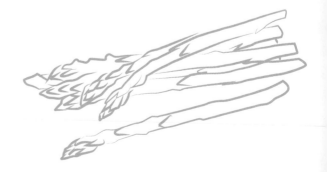

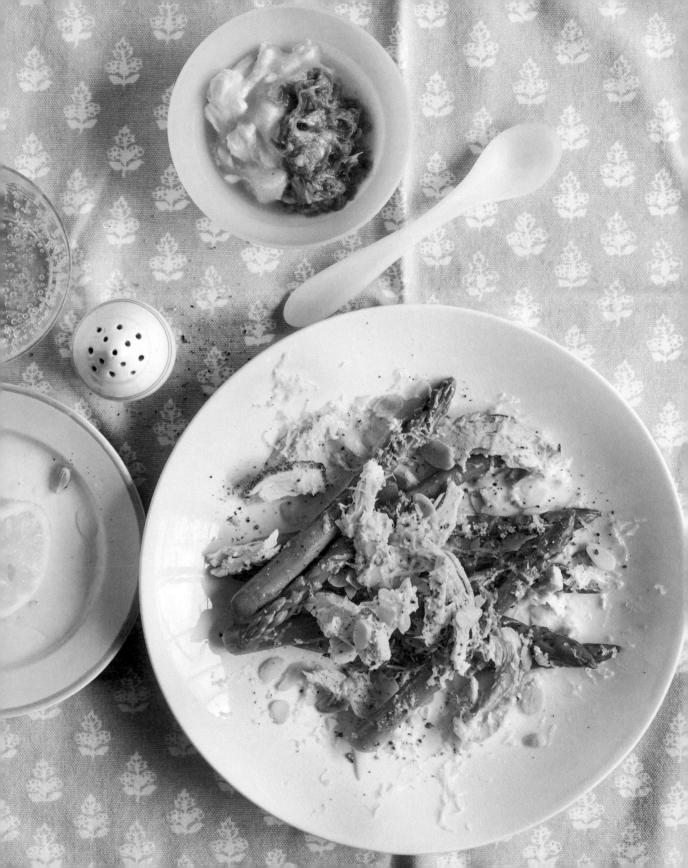

BABY GREEN BEANS WITH CORN
YOU TUNA & GREEN BEAN SALAD

Green beans are a nutritional hero, being an excellent source of vitamin K. They are a very good source of manganese, vitamin C, dietary fibre, folate, and vitamin B_2, and they also provide copper, vitamin B_1, chromium, magnesium, calcium, potassium, phosphorus, choline, vitamin A, niacin, iron, vitamin B_6, and vitamin E. Green beans have also been shown to contain valuable amounts of the mineral silicon, and in a form that makes it easier for the body to absorb this nutrient, which is needed for healthy bones and connective tissue.

Preparation time: 10 mins
Cooking time: 8-10 mins

TO PREPARE
50g green beans

FOR BABY
2 cubes frozen pear purée, thawed, or 2 tbsp (30ml) fresh pear purée

¹⁄₃ of the cooked green beans

2 tbsp (30ml) drained cooked corn, from an approximately 200g can or pouch with no added salt or sugar

FOR YOU
Serves 1
1 spring onion

A handful of cherry tomatoes

The remaining cooked green beans

The remaining drained corn

2 large handfuls of mixed salad leaves

A handful of pitted black olives

1 tbsp (15ml) capers (optional)

A small can (about 60g) good-quality tuna, drained if necessary

1 tbsp (15ml) olive oil

1 tbsp (15ml) balsamic vinegar

This is a great lunchtime salad: minimal prep, light but satisfying. The green beans provide plenty of nutrients, the tuna adds protein, the corn provides some light carbohydrate and more fibre, and the olives are a good source of healthy fats – a great all-round balanced dish.

Trim the ends from 50g green beans and place them in a pan of boiling water. Cover and cook for 8–10 minutes, until tender.

FOR BABY GREEN BEANS WITH CORN
Put the pear purée (which will mask the slight bitter taste of the beans) in a food processor with most of the beans. Reserve a few beans for your baby to hold while you are feeding him. Whizz together. Transfer to a bowl, add the corn and stir to combine.

FOR YOU TUNA & GREEN BEAN SALAD
Chop or snip the spring onion and halve the tomatoes. Place in the bowl with all the remaining ingredients and toss gently to coat with the oil and vinegar.

COOK'S TIP
You could hard-boil an egg while the beans are cooking. To do so, put an egg in a pan (it is best not to cook the egg in with the beans, since the exterior of the egg shell may not be that clean) with cold water and bring to a simmer. Once it is simmering, set a timer and boil the egg for 8 minutes. Drain and refill the pan with cold water, then leave the egg to cool until it is just warm (it is easier to peel off the shell when it is still slightly warm). Peel off the shell, chop the egg in half, then finely dice one half to stir into the green bean purée for your baby, and add the remainder to your salad.

BABY FRUITY FISHY LENTILS
YOU GREEN LENTIL SOUP

Green lentils are a good source of iron, but since it is in the form that is not so readily absorbed, combine lentils with a source of vitamin C (such as tomatoes and spinach), which aids iron absorption into the body. A lack of iron in the body can cause fatigue, which new mums can put down to lack of sleep. Lentils are also a great source of fibre, which prevents constipation and promotes a healthy digestive system.

Preparation time: 10 mins
Cooking time: 5-8 mins

TO PREPARE
A pouch of ready-to-eat green lentils

FOR BABY
1 small frozen white fish fillet

**2 cubes frozen apple purée
or 2 tbsp (30ml) fresh apple purée**

2 tbsp (30ml) of the lentils

1 tbsp (15ml) crème fraîche

2 cherry tomatoes

FOR YOU
Serves 2
1 tbsp (15ml) olive oil

2 spring onions

**1 tsp (5ml) garlic paste
or 1 garlic clove, crushed**

The remaining lentils
800ml low-salt vegetable stock

100g baby spinach leaves

2 tbsp (30ml) crème fraîche

6 cherry tomatoes

This is a hearty soup that both satisfies and nourishes. The lentils provide a good balance of protein, carbohydrate and fibre so you will feel energised all afternoon and shouldn't feel hungry again until dinnertime.

Take a pouch of ready-to-eat green lentils and microwave according to the packet instructions, then leave to stand. You could also use drained, rinsed canned lentils, or cook some dried lentils (be aware that the latter type require soaking and lengthy cooking).

FOR BABY FRUITY FISHY LENTILS
Place the fish and the frozen apple purée, if using, in a microwavable bowl and cook on High for 2 minutes. If you don't have a microwave, first thaw the fish, then put it in a small pan with 1cm water, cover, and cook over a medium heat for a few minutes, until the flesh is opaque and cooked through. Thaw the frozen apple purée separately if using this method. Mash the cooked fish into the thawed or fresh apple purée, then add the lentils and crème fraîche and use a fork to gently crush the lentils into the fish. Finely chop the cherry tomatoes and mix everything together.

FOR YOU GREEN LENTIL SOUP
Heat the oil in a pan. Use scissors to chop the spring onions, then add them to the pan with the garlic and cook for 2–3 minutes, until softened.

Add the remaining lentils and the stock and bring to the boil. Simmer for 5 minutes, then stir in the spinach leaves and crème fraîche.

Blend until smooth, then heat through. Chop the tomatoes and sprinkle on top.

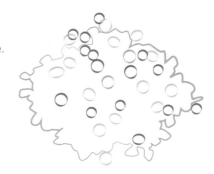

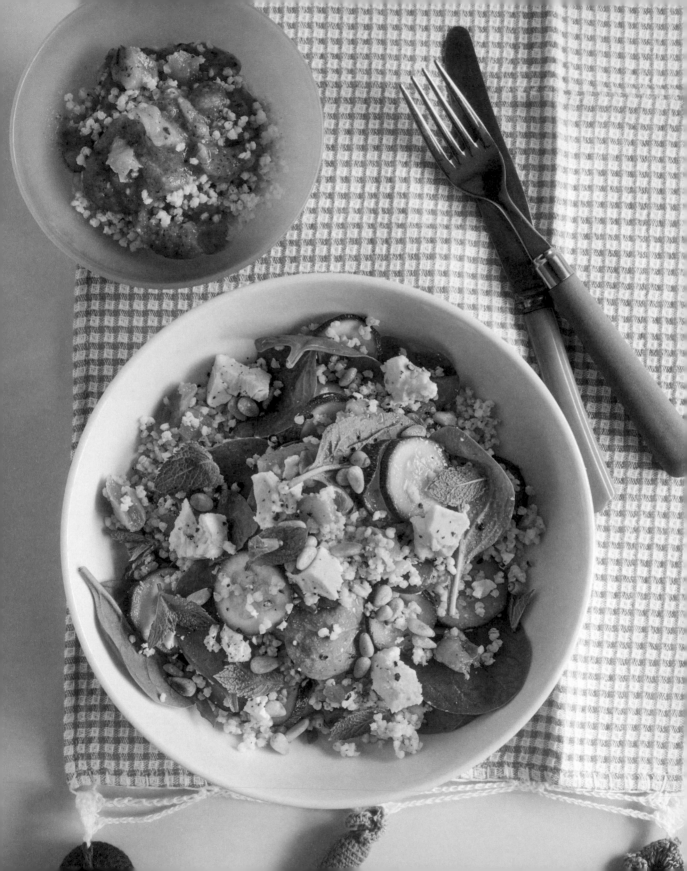

BABY MILLET & COURGETTE
YOU MILLET & FETA SALAD

Millet is a good wholegrain to introduce to your baby's diet. Research studies have linked it with a lower risk of developing childhood asthma and diabetes, and it provides plenty of fibre and good amounts of magnesium. Magnesium is needed for the healthy development of nerves and muscles.

Preparation time: 10 mins
Cooking time: 15-20 mins

TO PREPARE
100g millet

25 dried apricot pieces

400ml water or low-salt stock

1 courgette

FOR BABY
$^1/_3$ of the courgette slices

1 cube frozen apple purée, thawed, or 1 tbsp (15ml) fresh apple purée

3 tbsp (45ml) of the cooked millet

FOR YOU
Serves 1
The remaining cooked millet

The remaining cooked courgette

30g feta cheese

A couple of fresh mint leaves

A large handful of baby spinach leaves

1 tbsp (15ml) pine nuts

Millet has a low GI so will release its energy slowly. This can be beneficial if you are planning to catch up on your sleep while your baby takes his afternoon nap; eating foods with a high GI will disrupt your blood-sugar levels, which can interfere with sleeping. As it's so important to grab sleep when you can, avoid anything that will have this effect.

Place the millet and apricots in a pan and pour in the water or stock. Bring to the boil, turn down the heat and simmer for 15–20 minutes, until the water has been absorbed and the millet is fluffy.

While the millet is cooking, slice a courgette and steam it for 6–8 minutes.

FOR BABY MILLET & COURGETTE
Place the apple purée in a bowl and add one-third of the courgette slices. Gently mash together, then stir in the cooked millet.

FOR YOU MILLET & FETA SALAD
Put the millet and courgette in a bowl. Dice the feta and tear the mint leaves and mix into the millet with the spinach, then scatter over the pine nuts. For extra flavour, toast the pine nuts by dry-frying them in a frying pan for 1–2 minutes, tossing frequently, until golden.

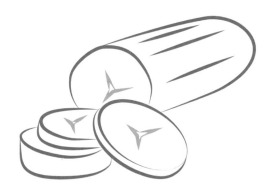

BABY CREAMY LENTIL DHAL
YOU SPICY DHAL

The star nutrient of red lentils is the mineral molybdenum, which is needed for a number of important biological functions in the body, such as supporting the nervous system, hormone regulation and energy production. Lentils are a very good source of dietary fibre, copper, phosphorus, folate and manganese. In addition, they provide iron, protein, zinc, potassium, and B vitamins. They are also very easy to use, since unlike most types of dried lentil red lentils require no soaking and cook relatively quickly, meaning they are a very economical and healthy store cupboard ingredient.

Preparation time: 5 mins
Cooking time: 25-30 mins

TO PREPARE
A drizzle of olive oil

1 spring onion

4 frozen cubes butternut squash purée, thawed, or 4 tbsp (60ml) fresh butternut squash purée

4 frozen cubes sweet potato purée, thawed, or 4 tbsp (60ml) fresh sweet potato purée

1 tsp (5ml) ground cumin

100g dried red lentils

400ml low-salt stock

1 tomato

FOR BABY
2 tbsp (30ml) of the dhal

1 tbsp (15ml) soft white cheese

Toast fingers, for dipping

FOR YOU
Serves 1
The remaining Dhal

A few drops of chilli sauce or ½ tsp (2.5ml) chilli powder or hot smoked paprika

Fresh coriander leaves

Toasted wholemeal pitta or small naan

A dollop of mango chutney

Sometimes you need something that you know is healthy but seems indulgent. This is it: dipping toasted pitta into spicy dhal with dollops of mango chutney is heaven!

Heat the oil in a pan. Use scissors to chop the spring onion, then add to the pan and cook for 2–3 minutes, until soft. Add the butternut squash and sweet potato purées and the ground cumin and cook for 1 minute.

Add the lentils and stock, bring to the boil, then simmer for 20 minutes, stirring occasionally. Chop the tomato and add it to the mixture 5 minutes before the end. The dhal will be fairly smooth without blending, but if you prefer it silky smooth then blend it to your preferred texture.

FOR BABY CREAMY LENTIL DHAL
Mix together the dhal and cheese. Give your baby some toast fingers to dip in the mixture.

FOR YOU SPICY DHAL
Spice up the remaining dhal with a few drops of chilli sauce, chilli powder or hot smoked paprika and sprinkle on some fresh coriander leaves. Eat with a toasted wholemeal pitta or small naan and a dollop of mango chutney.

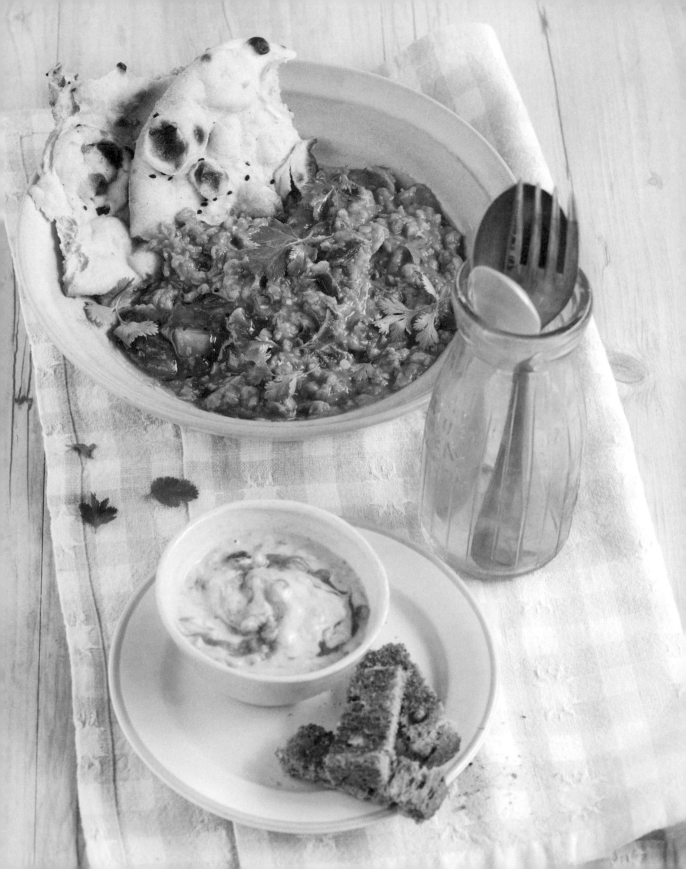

BABY RAISIN & CARROT BULGUR

YOU TABBOULEH

This is another wholegrain to introduce into your baby's diet. It does contain gluten, so it should be introduced from six months onwards. It has a low GI and plenty of fibre, and its main vitamin is niacin – needed for growth and development – while its main mineral is magnesium – needed for good bone and muscle health.

Preparation time: 10 mins
Cooking time: 20-30 mins

TO PREPARE
200ml boiling water

1 low-salt stock cube

75g bulgur

1 tbsp (15ml) sultanas

FOR BABY
1 carrot

2 tbsp (30ml) of the cooked bulgur

FOR YOU
Serves 1

The remaining carrot

The remaining bulgur

1 tbsp (15ml) pumpkin seeds

1 tbsp (15ml) hazelnuts

Juice from ½ lemon

1 tbsp (15ml) rapeseed oil

30g feta cheese

Ground black pepper

A handful of mint leaves

Bulgur is so versatile it pretty much goes with anything. It's delicious with feta and mint, but you could also use chicken, chickpeas, avocado or edamame. It has a lovely nutty taste that partners well with nuts and seeds, and you could use any herbs you have to hand to add vibrancy and flavour.

Measure the boiling water into a heatproof bowl, then add the stock cube and stir to dissolve. Add the bulgur and sultanas, cover the bowl with cling film and leave for 20–30 minutes for the liquid to be absorbed. Once absorbed, run a fork through the grains to separate. Leave to cool.

FOR BABY RAISIN & CARROT BULGUR
While the bulgur is soaking, peel the carrot and chop it in half. Finely dice one half, place in a pan of boiling water and cook for 8–10 minutes, until tender. Alternatively, microwave the carrots with a drop of water on High for 2 minutes, give them a stir, then microwave for a further 1–2 minutes, until tender.

Put the bulgur in a bowl and stir in the cooked carrot. Mix together, and gently mash the carrot and raisins into the bulgur.

FOR YOU TABBOULEH
Grate the remaining carrot into the bulgur and add the pumpkin seeds, hazelnuts, lemon juice and rapeseed oil. Stir to combine well, then crumble in the feta and season with black pepper. Mix gently to combine. Tear the mint leaves and scatter over the top.

BABY BUTTER BEAN MASH
YOU FAGIOLI

Nutritionally, butter beans are quite similar to chickpeas in that they are a good source of protein and fibre. The latter helps to maintain even blood-sugar levels and aids digestion, helping to prevent constipation. The main nutrients are folate, iron and manganese.

Preparation time: 10 mins
Cooking time: 2-3 mins

TO PREPARE
400g can of butter beans

FOR BABY
A pat of butter

1 spring onion

2 tbsp (30ml) of the butter beans

1 tbsp (15ml) soft white cheese

¹/₃ of a can (about 120g) of good-quality tuna in spring water or oil, drained if necessary

FOR YOU
Serves 1
1 garlic clove

1 spring onion

2 tomatoes

The remaining butter beans

The remaining tuna

Juice of ½ lemon

1 tbsp (15ml) white wine vinegar

A handful of parsley leaves

Ground black pepper

This is a lovely light dish that you can make in minutes. It's packed full of protein and fibre so should keep you going through even the busiest afternoon.

Rinse and drain a 400g can of butter beans.

FOR BABY BUTTER BEAN MASH
Heat the butter in a pan. Use scissors to snip a spring onion, then add to the pan and cook for 2–3 minutes, until softened.

Meanwhile, mash the butter beans with a fork. Add to the onion, mix well and heat through. Stir in the cheese and the tuna and warm through.

FOR YOU FAGIOLI
Peel and finely chop the garlic and place it in a bowl. Chop the spring onion and tomatoes and add to the bowl along with the butter beans and tuna.

Add the lemon juice and vinegar and toss together, then tear the parsley leaves and scatter over the top. Season to taste with black pepper.

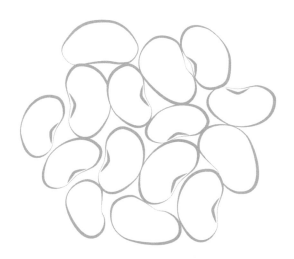

BABY QUINOA PILAF
YOU QUINOA SALAD

Quinoa is higher in protein than most other grains. Like all wholegrains, it has a low GI and provides plenty of fibre. It is a good source of B vitamins and a particularly good source of manganese, which is needed by the body as an antioxidant that protects cells from damage.

Preparation time: 10 mins
Cooking time: 15-20 mins

TO PREPARE
200ml boiling water

1 low-salt stock cube

A drizzle of olive oil

75g dried quinoa

3 cubes frozen butternut squash purée or 3 tbsp (45ml) fresh butternut squash purée

1 skinless chicken breast

Ground black pepper

FOR BABY
1/3 of the cooked chicken breast

2 tbsp (30ml) of the cooked quinoa

FOR YOU
Serves 1
1 spring onion

The remaining quinoa

1 tbsp (15ml) dried cranberries

1 tbsp (15ml) pecan nuts

2 handfuls of baby spinach leaves or rocket

The remaining chicken

A handful of parsley leaves

A drizzle of olive oil

A drizzle of balsamic vinegar

This is a protein-packed salad that will keep you feeling full all afternoon. It is also extremely versatile – you can swap most of the ingredients for whatever fruit, nuts and herbs you have to hand, and you can make it vegetarian by using chopped hard-boiled egg or some feta or goat's cheese in place of the chicken breast.

Measure the boiling water into a heatproof bowl, then add the stock cube and stir to dissolve.

Heat the olive oil in a pan and add the quinoa. Stir to coat the grains in the oil, then add the hot stock, bring to the boil and simmer for 15 minutes.

Add the frozen butternut squash purée, if using, and heat for a further 5 minutes, or add the fresh purée after the quinoa has been cooking for 20 minutes. Stir the purée through the quinoa and ensure it is heated through.

While the quinoa is simmering, preheat the oven to 200ºC (Gas 6). Place a skinless chicken breast in a baking dish, drizzle with olive oil, season lightly with a little pepper and cook in the oven for 20 minutes.

FOR BABY QUINOA PILAF
Finely dice the chicken, then stir it through the quinoa and serve.

FOR BABY QUINOA SALAD
Use scissors to chop the spring onion, then add it to the remaining quinoa. Stir in the cranberries, nuts and spinach or rocket.

Shred the chicken and place it on top. Tear the parsley leaves and scatter on top, then drizzle over a little oil and vinegar.

QUICK QUINOA

If you don't have time to cook raw quinoa, you can use a pouch of ready-cooked quinoa, or a mixture of brown basmati rice and quinoa. These pouches take just 2 minutes to heat in the microwave and are extremely convenient, albeit more expensive.

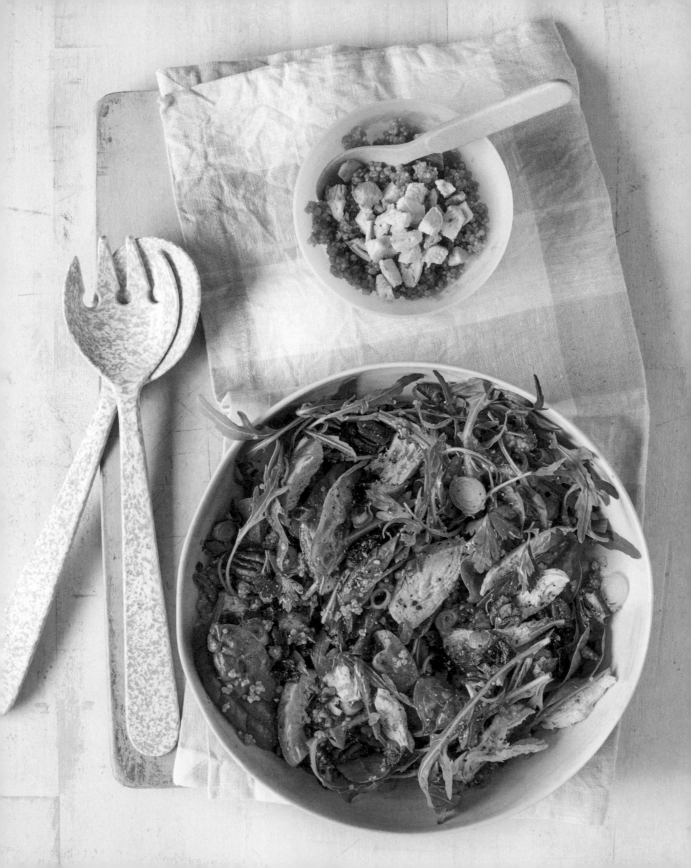

BABY BABY HUMMUS
YOU HUMMUS, APPLE & AVOCADO WRAP

Chickpeas contain a good balance of carbohydrate, protein and fibre and so make a great basis for a healthy meal. They have many vitamins and minerals; in particular they are a good source of folate and iron, both of which are needed for healthy blood.

Preparation time: 10 mins
Cooking time: 0 mins

TO PREPARE
400g can of chickpeas

FOR BABY
3 cubes frozen sweet potato purée, thawed, or 3 tbsp (45ml) fresh sweet potato purée

2 tbsp (30ml) of the chickpeas

1 tbsp (15ml) plain Greek yogurt

Slices of apple and avocado, and plain rice cakes, for dipping

FOR YOU
Serves 1
The remaining chickpeas

1 tsp (5ml) garlic paste or 1 garlic clove, crushed

2 tbsp (30ml) plain Greek yogurt

1 tbsp (15ml) tahini

Juice of 1 lemon

1 tbsp (15ml) olive oil

A handful of fresh coriander leaves

1 wholegrain wrap

The remaining apple and avocado

Shop-bought hummus is fine, but if you have the time it's worth making your own as you can get the flavour and texture exactly as you like. Once made, it will last in the fridge for 3–4 days and you can use any leftovers as a dip for veg sticks or to spread on oatcakes for a healthy snack.

Rinse and drain a 400g can of chickpeas.

FOR BABY BABY HUMMUS
Mash together the sweet potato purée and chickpeas, then stir in the Greek yogurt. Give your baby slices of apple and avocado and plain rice cakes to dip in.

FOR YOU HUMMUS, APPLE & AVOCADO WRAP
Tip the remaining chickpeas into a food processor. Add the garlic, yogurt, tahini, lemon juice, oil and half the coriander leaves and whizz together.

Spread the hummus over the wrap, then add slices of the apple and avocado, sprinkle on the rest of the coriander leaves and wrap up.

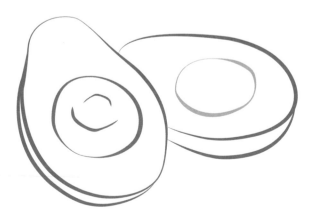

BABY SARDINE MASH
YOU SARDINE DIP

Sardines are an oily fish, so are a good source of omega-3 fats, needed for your baby's developing brain. They are also a good source of selenium and vitamin D. Sardine bones are soft and edible, which makes them a good source of calcium, which combined with the vitamin D make sardines a good choice for healthy bones.

Preparation time: 5 mins
Cooking time: 10 mins

TO PREPARE
2 cans of sardines in oil
(about 100–120g each)

3 tbsp (45ml) soft white cheese

1 tbsp (15ml) lemon juice

FOR BABY
1 medium-sized potato or sweet potato

A pat of butter

1 tbsp (15ml) of the sardine mixture

FOR YOU
Serves 1
The remaining sardine mixture

Oatcakes, or celery and carrot sticks

If you've never been tempted to open a can of sardines, this recipe will change your mind. It's super-quick and easy and goes perfectly with the oatcakes.

Drain the oil from the sardines and place in a food processor. Add the soft white cheese and lemon juice and whizz together to form a smooth paste.

FOR BABY SARDINE MASH
Peel and chop the potato or sweet potato, then add to a pan of boiling water. Cook for 10 minutes until tender, then drain and transfer to a bowl. Add the butter, mash until smooth, then stir in the sardine mixture.

FOR YOU SARDINE DIP
Simply serve the sardine mixture with the oatcakes or vegetable sticks and get dipping.

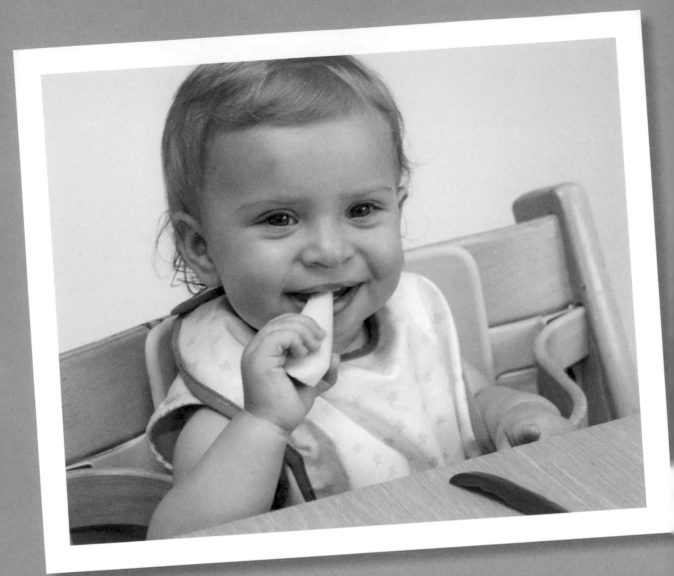

STAGE 2
DINNERS

As your baby starts to enjoy a wider range of food you should introduce foods with more flavour and texture, this includes different wholegrains and protein foods like meat and fish. These recipes each introduce one new ingredient with some familiar ingredients that hopefully your baby is already eating happily. The idea is that this will gently nudge them to the next stage of enjoying family meals.

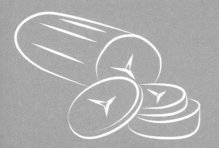
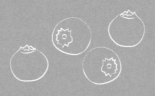
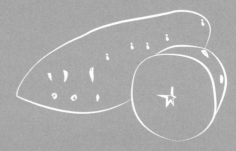

BABY CARIBBEAN BEANS & RICE
YOU SPICY TOFU WITH BEANS & RICE

Try to include kidney beans in your baby's and your own diet on a regular basis as they have numerous health benefits. Not only do they help to balance blood-sugar levels while supplying slow-burning energy, but they also provide protein for growth and development and much-needed iron to boost body stores and keep blood healthy.

Preparation time: 10 mins
Cooking time: 15-20 mins

TO PREPARE
A small can (about 300g) kidney beans in water

A drizzle of olive oil

2 spring onions

1 tsp (5ml) dried oregano

½ tsp (2.5ml) paprika

250g cooked brown basmati rice (a microwave pouch is most convenient)

FOR BABY
2 tbsp (30ml) of the cooked brown basmati rice

1 tbsp (15ml) of the kidney bean mixture

1 tbsp (15ml) coconut milk

FOR YOU
Serves 1
100g tofu

1 tsp (5ml) jerk seasoning

A drizzle of vegetable oil

50g pak choi

50g long-stem broccoli

2 tbsp (30ml) cashew nuts

The remaining cooked brown basmati rice

The remaining kidney bean mixture

2 tbsp (30ml) coconut milk

This dish is a great choice for when you are short on time but need a substantial meal. The tofu cooks in minutes and is the perfect blank canvas for the lovely Caribbean flavours of the jerk spice and coconut milk. It also holds its own in the protein stakes, containing just as much high-quality protein as non-vegetarian sources.

Drain and rinse the kidney beans. Heat the olive oil in a pan and use scissors to chop in the spring onions. Add the oregano and paprika and cook for 2–3 minutes, until softened. Add the kidney beans and cook for another 3–4 minutes. Cook or heat the rice according to the packet instructions.

FOR BABY CARIBBEAN BEANS & RICE
Put the rice in a small pan and add the kidney bean mixture. Use a fork to gently mash the beans. Add the coconut milk, stir well and gently heat through. You could add 1 tsp (5ml) ground cumin to add more flavour, if you like.

FOR YOU SPICY TOFU WITH BEANS & RICE
Dice the tofu and place it in a bowl, then add the jerk seasoning and toss to coat.

Heat the oil in a wok, then add the tofu and stir-fry for 6–8 minutes. Add the pak choi, broccoli and cashew nuts after 3–4 minutes, then the rice and the bean mixture.

Stir in the coconut milk and cook for 2 minutes to heat everything through.

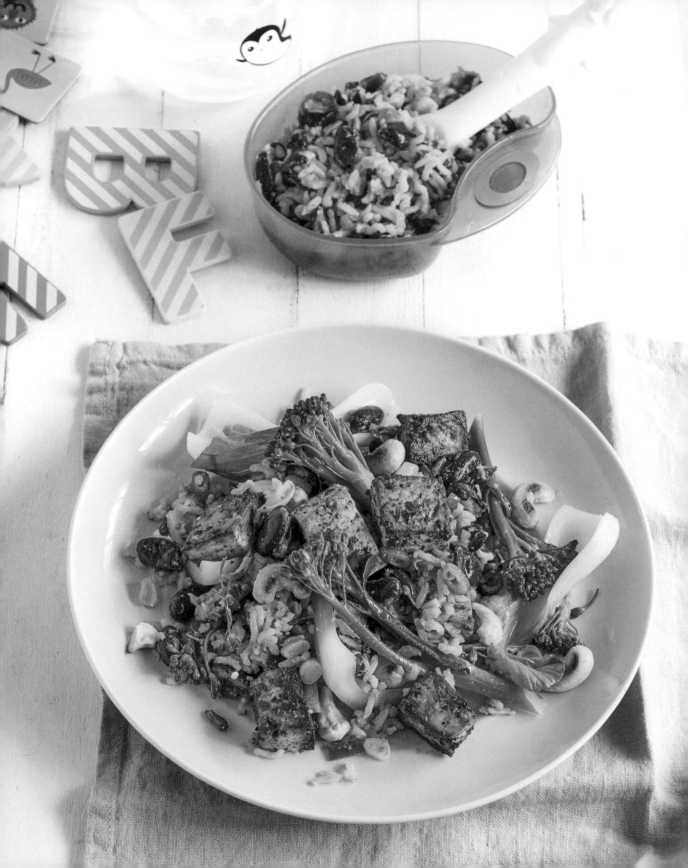

BABY MUSHROOM BARLEY
YOU MACKEREL & MUSHROOM BARLEY

It's a great idea to get your baby to experience different kinds of grain other than refined types of wheat and, as cereal grains go, barley is a winner when it comes to good nutrition. This centuries-old grain is packed with the type of fibre that helps to balance blood-sugar levels and also contains important vitamins and minerals, including B vitamins, selenium, iron, magnesium, zinc, phosphorus and copper.

Preparation time: 15 mins
Cooking time: 40 mins

TO PREPARE
75g barley

A drizzle of olive oil

5 mushrooms

A pat of butter

1 tsp (5ml) garlic paste
or 1 clove garlic, crushed

FOR BABY
2 tbsp (30ml) of the barley mixture

1 tbsp (15ml) of the cooked mushrooms

1 tbsp (15ml) ricotta

1 tbsp (15ml) snipped chives

FOR YOU
Serves 1
50g green beans

2 thin smoked mackerel fillets

The remaining cooked mushrooms

The remaining cooked barley

1 spring onion

A handful of baby spinach leaves

A handful of chives

This makes a delicious supper; the barley has a lovely nutty flavour that goes well with the mushrooms. Mushrooms are a great source of fibre – a type that helps lower cholesterol levels – as well as the minerals selenium and copper, and B vitamins. The smoked mackerel counts towards your recommended weekly oily fish intake.

Put the barley in a pan, cover with cold water and bring to the boil. Simmer for about 40 minutes, until the barley is soft and tender (or you can remove 50g after 30 minutes if you prefer it to be al dente). Drain and drizzle with the olive oil.

While the barley is cooking, finely chop the mushrooms. Heat the butter in a pan, add the garlic and the mushrooms and sauté for 5 minutes.

FOR BABY MUSHROOM BARLEY
Put the barley in a bowl, then stir in the mushrooms and ricotta. Sprinkle with some snipped chives.

FOR YOU MACKEREL & MUSHROOM BARLEY
Steam or boil the green beans for 5 minutes, then drain and roughly chop.

Flake the mackerel flesh away from the skin.

Mix the mushrooms into the cooked barley.

Use scissors to chop the spring onion and add to the barley along with the spinach leaves, green beans and the mackerel. Toss well together and sprinkle with some snipped chives.

STORING MUSHROOMS
Instead of storing your mushrooms in the fridge, keep them on the windowsill to expose them to sunlight: this will build up their vitamin D content before you eat them.

BABY SWEET POTATO SALMON
YOU SALMON WITH WILD-RICE HERBY SALAD

Salmon is a valuable source of two important omega-3 fats. While breast or formula feeding, your baby will receive a good supply of these, but as weaning starts it is important to find good food sources to continue her intake. Oily fish such as salmon, sardines and mackerel contain the most, so aim to offer a type of oily fish once or twice a week.

Preparation time: 15 mins
Cooking time: 20 mins

TO PREPARE
2 large salmon fillets

A drizzle of olive oil

200g plain Greek yogurt

Juice of ½ lemon

A handful of chopped dill

FOR BABY
3 cubes frozen sweet potato purée, thawed, or 45ml (3 tbsp) fresh sweet potato purée

50g of the flaked salmon

2 tsp (10ml) of the yogurt mixture

FOR YOU
Serves 2
250g cooked brown basmati and wild rice (a microwave pouch is most convenient)

100g mangetout

4 spears of long-stem broccoli

50g frozen peas

½ cucumber

6 cherry tomatoes

1 avocado

A handful each of fresh basil, coriander, parsley and mint

The remaining flaked salmon

The remaining yogurt mixture

The omega-3 fats in oily fish can help to improve mood and reduce the risk of depression, including postnatal depression. These clever fats also look after your heart and joints by reducing inflammation and help to lower the risk of developing cancer and type 2 diabetes.

Preheat the oven to 200°C (Gas 6). Place the salmon fillets skin side down in a roasting tin and drizzle with olive oil. Bake for 20 minutes.

Meanwhile, mix the Greek yogurt with the lemon juice and chopped dill. Remove the salmon from the oven and flake the flesh into a bowl.

FOR BABY SWEET POTATO SALMON
Put the sweet potato purée in a small pan. Add the flaked salmon and gently heat together. Transfer to a bowl and swirl through the yogurt mixture.

FOR YOU SALMON WITH WILD-RICE HERBY SALAD
Put the cooked rice in a large bowl. Steam or boil the mangetout, broccoli and peas for 5 minutes, until slightly cooked but with bite.

Roughly chop the cucumber, tomatoes and avocado and tear the herbs, then add to the rice. Chop the broccoli and add to the rice with the mangetout and peas.

Toss everything together. Place the salmon flakes on top and drizzle with a few spoonfuls of the yogurt. Serve the rest on the side.

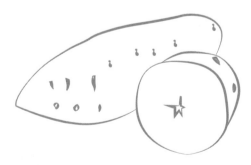

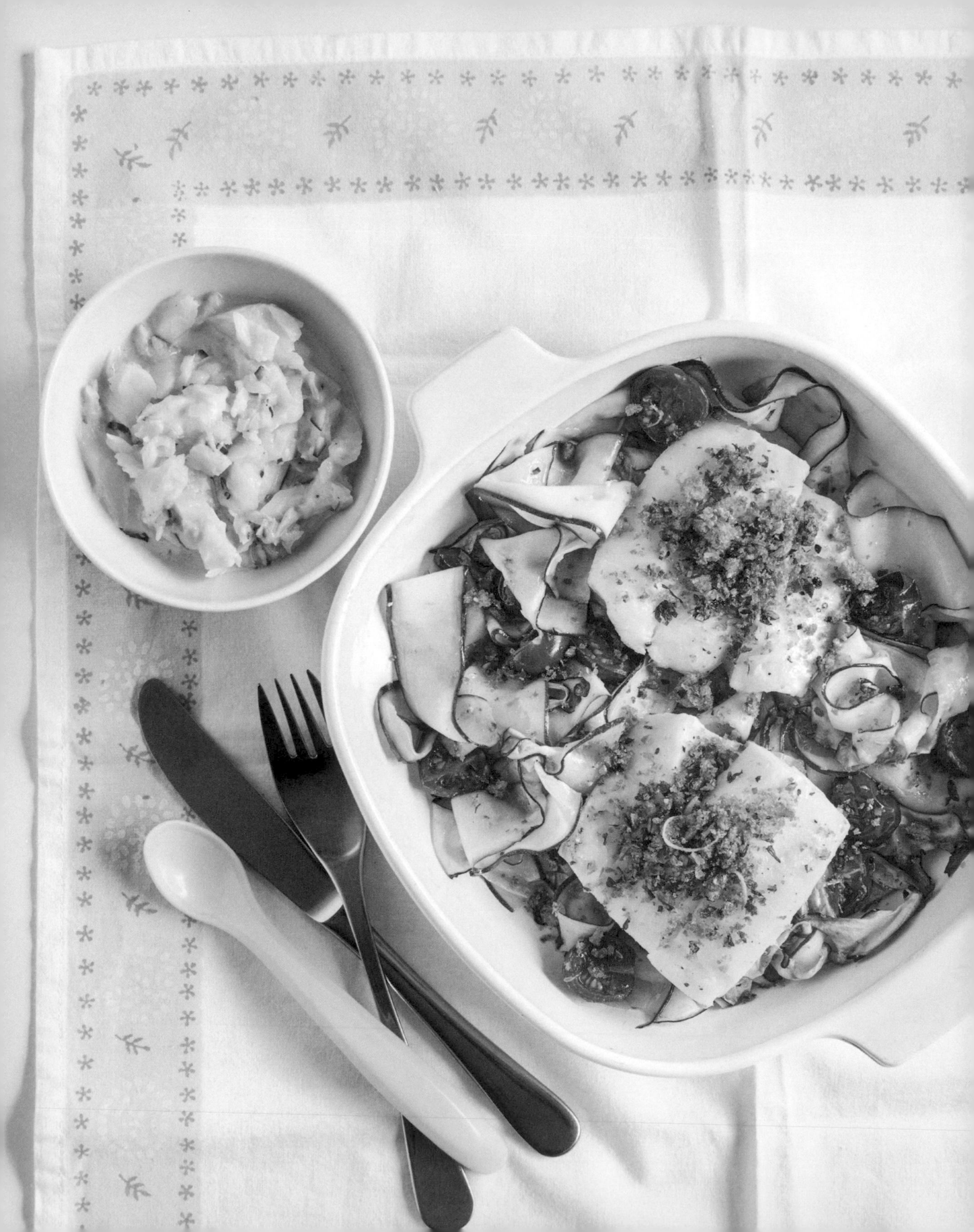

BABY CHEESY COURGETTE FISH
YOU HERB-CRUSTED FISH

Sustainable white fish such as pollack, hake, coley, plaice and lemon sole are a great addition to your baby's diet as they provide texture and lumpiness to a dish, but the lumps are soft and easy to eat. White fish is a good source of protein and extremely high in selenium and iodine. It's a good idea to encourage your baby to eat fish on a regular basis so they get used to it and start to enjoy it. Like selenium, iodine intakes are generally low and if you don't encourage your baby to eat fish there are few other sources that can provide it.

Preparation time: 15 mins
Cooking time: 20 mins

TO PREPARE
2 courgettes
8 cherry tomatoes
3 skinless white fish fillets
A drizzle of olive oil
Juice of 1 lemon

FOR BABY
2 strips of the roasted courgette
1 of the roasted white fish fillets
1 tbsp (15ml) crème fraîche
A handful of grated cheese

FOR YOU
Serves 2
The remaining roasted white fish fillets
1 fresh red chilli
1 garlic clove, peeled
Grated rind of the lemon
2 slices of wholemeal bread
A handful of parsley leaves
A pat of butter

The breadcrumb topping is a simple way to give this dish an extra flavour punch. It's a light, high-protein supper for those days when you feel you might have over-indulged on tea and cake with your new parent friends.

Preheat the oven to 180ºC (Gas 4). Thinly slice the courgettes lengthways and halve the cherry tomatoes. Place in a roasting tin. Place the fish fillets on top and drizzle with olive oil and lemon juice. Bake for 20 minutes, or until the fish is opaque and flakes easily.

FOR BABY CHEESY COURGETTE FISH
Finely chop the courgette and place in a small pan. Add the fish and break it apart by mashing it with a fork. Stir in the crème fraîche and grated cheese and gently heat though until the cheese has melted into the crème fraîche.

FOR YOU HERB-CRUSTED FISH
While the fish is baking, split the chilli, remove the seeds and roughly chop the flesh. Peel the garlic. Place the chilli, garlic, lemon zest, bread and parsley in a food processor and whizz together.

Heat a pat of butter and fry the breadcrumb mixture for 3–4 minutes, stirring frequently, until golden. Serve on top of the fish once it is cooked.

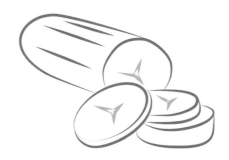

BABY CHINESE CHICKEN
YOU CHICKEN LAKSA

Chicken is a great source of B vitamins which have various functions in the body including boosting immunity and cell growth, keeping nerve and blood cells healthy. It also contains iron and zinc.

Preparation time: 15 mins
Cooking time: 30 mins

TO PREPARE
200g chicken breast

A pinch of Chinese five spice

A drizzle of olive oil

100g green beans

FOR BABY
2 tbsp (30ml) of the cooked chicken

2 tbsp (30ml) of the cooked green beans

2 cubes frozen butternut squash purée, thawed, or 2 tbsp (30ml) fresh butternut squash purée

2 cubes frozen sweet potato purée, thawed, or 2 tbsp (30ml) fresh sweet potato purée

FOR YOU
Serves 2

A drizzle of olive oil

1 tsp (5ml) chilli paste

1 tsp (5ml) ginger paste

4 spring onions

1 red pepper

The remaining cooked green beans

The remaining cooked chicken

800ml hot low-salt chicken or vegetable stock

2 large handfuls of baby spinach leaves

A pack (about 300g) of fresh glass noodles

1 tbsp (15ml) soy sauce

1 tbsp (15ml) fish sauce

Juice of 1 lime

A few fresh coriander leaves

A laksa is a cross between a soup and a stew, so it's instantly filling and satisfying and doesn't need anything else to go with it. The glass noodles provide the carbohydrate, the chicken provides the protein and there is enough veg to count as three of your five a day.

Dice the chicken breast and sprinkle with the Chinese five spice. Heat a drizzle of olive oil in a frying pan, add the chicken and fry for 10 minutes, until the chicken is thoroughly cooked through. While the chicken is cooking, steam or boil the green beans.

FOR BABY CHINESE CHICKEN
This dish contains small lumps of chicken and green beans and is a step on from the coarser purées your baby may previously have been eating. The butternut squash and sweet potato purées will help him swallow the small lumps but you may need to use a hand-held blender to give the dish a quick whizz if he doesn't like the lumps to begin with.

Finely chop the chicken and green beans.

Put the butternut squash and sweet potato purées in a small pan, add the chicken and beans and gently heat everything through. Stir well to coat the chicken and beans in the purée.

FOR YOU CHICKEN LAKSA
Heat the oil in a frying pan, then add the chilli and ginger pastes. Use scissors to chop in the spring onions.

Deseed and slice the pepper and slice the green beans, then add them to the pan. Cook for 3–4 minutes, until the spring onion and pepper are softened.

Add the remaining chicken, stock, spinach leaves and glass noodles. Bring to the boil, then add the soy sauce, fish sauce and lime juice and simmer for 4 minutes.

Serve topped with a few coriander leaves.

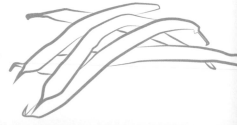

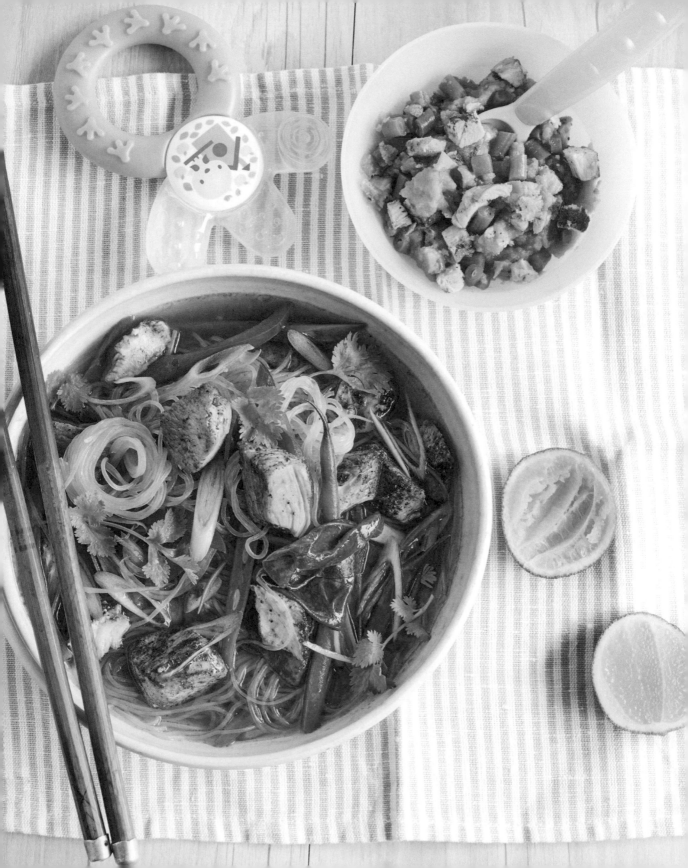

BABY TURKEY WITH APRICOT & SPINACH

YOU SPICY TURKEY & APRICOT MEATBALLS

You might think turkey is not much different to chicken, but nutritionally there are some significant distinctions that do make it a worthwhile addition to your baby's diet. Both are a great source of easy-to-digest protein and both supply B vitamins needed to keep your little one energised, but turkey is richer in the minerals selenium and chromium. Selenium, a powerful antioxidant, can often be in short supply in the diet so turkey is a convenient way to improve intake. Chromium keeps blood-sugar levels healthy as it is needed to balance insulin.

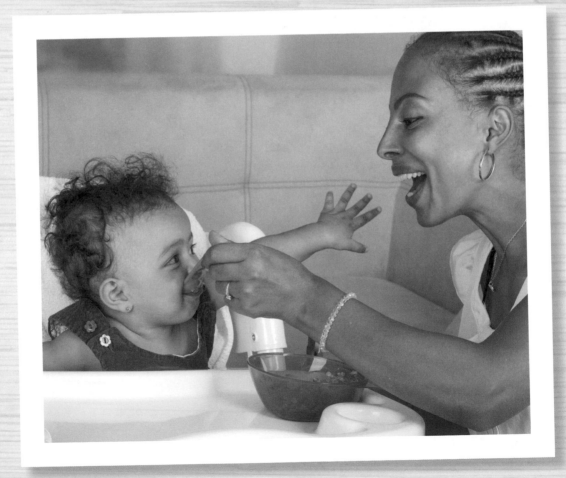

Preparation time: 20 mins
Cooking time: 25 mins

TO PREPARE
200g turkey mince

2 spring onions

50g dried ready-to-eat apricots

FOR BABY
A drizzle of olive oil

2 tbsp (30ml) of the turkey mixture

A handful of chopped spinach leaves

25g couscous

3 tbsp (45ml) boiling water

A squeeze of lemon juice

FOR YOU
Serves 2
The remaining turkey mixture

1 tsp (5ml) chilli paste

1 tsp (5ml) garlic paste or 1 garlic clove, crushed

1 tsp (5ml) lemongrass paste

Salt and ground black pepper

1 egg

1 tbsp (15ml) olive oil

60g couscous

7 tbsp (105ml) hot low-salt chicken or vegetable stock

Juice of ½ lemon

1 green pepper

1 pack (about 110g) pomegranate seeds

1 tbsp (15ml) pine nuts

A handful of fresh coriander leaves

These meatballs contain a lovely blend of spice, heat and natural sweetness and are a good choice if you need to unwind after a busy day as the turkey contains the amino acid tryptophan, which is needed for the production of serotonin – aka the body's 'happy hormone' – that can help you relax and aids sleep.

Place the turkey mince in a bowl. Use scissors to finely chop in the spring onions and dried apricots, and stir to combine.

FOR BABY TURKEY WITH APRICOT & SPINACH
Heat the olive oil in a pan, add the turkey mixture and spinach leaves and cook gently for 6–8 minutes.

Meanwhile, place the couscous in a bowl and add the boiling water and lemon juice. Cover and allow to stand for 5 minutes, then fluff the grains with a fork.

Stir the turkey mixture through the couscous.

FOR YOU SPICY TURKEY & APRICOT MEATBALLS
Put the turkey mince in a bowl and add the chilli, garlic and lemongrass. Season with a pinch of salt and plenty of black pepper, then stir in the egg.

Use your hands to combine the mixture, then form into 10–12 evenly sized meatballs. Dampen your hands if you find the mixture is sticking to them.

Heat the oil in a frying pan, add the meatballs and fry, turning frequently, for 15 minutes, until browned and cooked through.

Meanwhile, put the couscous in a bowl with the hot stock and lemon juice, cover and allow to stand for 5 minutes. Fluff up with a fork.

Deseed and finely chop the green pepper, then add it to the couscous with the pomegranate seeds and pine nuts and stir to combine. Sprinkle over the coriander leaves and serve with the meatballs.

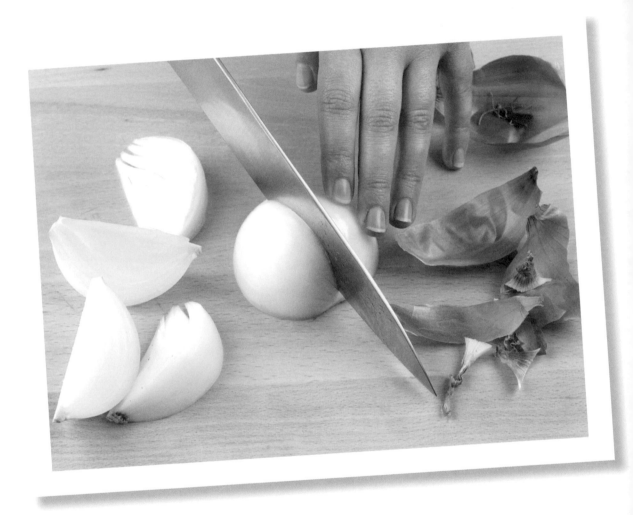

BABY MINCED BEEF WITH PEAS

YOU KEEMA

Just like lamb, beef is a rich source of protein, easily absorbed iron, selenium, zinc and vitamin B_{12}. Choose good-quality beef that has been grass fed, as this improves the content of healthy fats, vitamin E and beta-carotene. Iron is particularly important for preventing feelings of lethargy and fatigue.

Preparation time: 5 mins
Cooking time: 35 mins

TO PREPARE

1 onion

1 garlic clove

A drizzle of olive oil

250g beef mince

1 small can (about 225g) chopped tomatoes

100g frozen peas

FOR BABY

2 tbsp (30ml) of the beef mixture

2 cubes frozen sweet potato purée, thawed, or 2 tbsp (30ml) sweet potato purée

FOR YOU

Serves 2

1 tsp (5ml) chilli paste

1 tsp (5ml) ginger paste

2 tbsp (30ml) garam masala

Salt and ground black pepper

The remaining beef mixture

2 tbsp (30ml) plain Greek yogurt

A handful of coriander leaves

Roti or other flatbreads, to serve

Here's a really quick curry that takes minimal effort and will be ready before one can be delivered. As tempting as it is to resort to a takeaway when you're dog tired, just remember the quality of the ingredients will never be a match for your own home-made versions and so will do little to nourish your body.

Peel the onion and garlic, place in a food processor and whizz to finely chop.

Heat a drizzle of olive oil in a heavy pan, then add the onion and garlic and cook for 1–2 minutes. Add the beef mince and cook for a further 2–3 minutes, until brown.

Stir in the chopped tomatoes, then simmer, uncovered, for 20 minutes. Stir in the frozen peas and cook for a further 10 minutes.

FOR BABY MINCED BEEF WITH PEAS

Put the beef mixture and sweet potato purée in a small pan and gently heat through.

FOR YOU KEEMA

Stir the chilli, ginger and garam masala into the remaining beef mixture while it is still in the pan, season with a pinch of salt and plenty of black pepper and continue to cook for 1–2 minutes to release the flavours.

Reduce the heat, then stir in the yogurt and gently heat through. Sprinkle over the coriander leaves and serve with roti or other flatbreads.

FREEZING FLATBREADS

You can freeze ready-made flatbreads, then simply put them in the oven from frozen and cook or grill for a few minutes, according to the packet instructions.

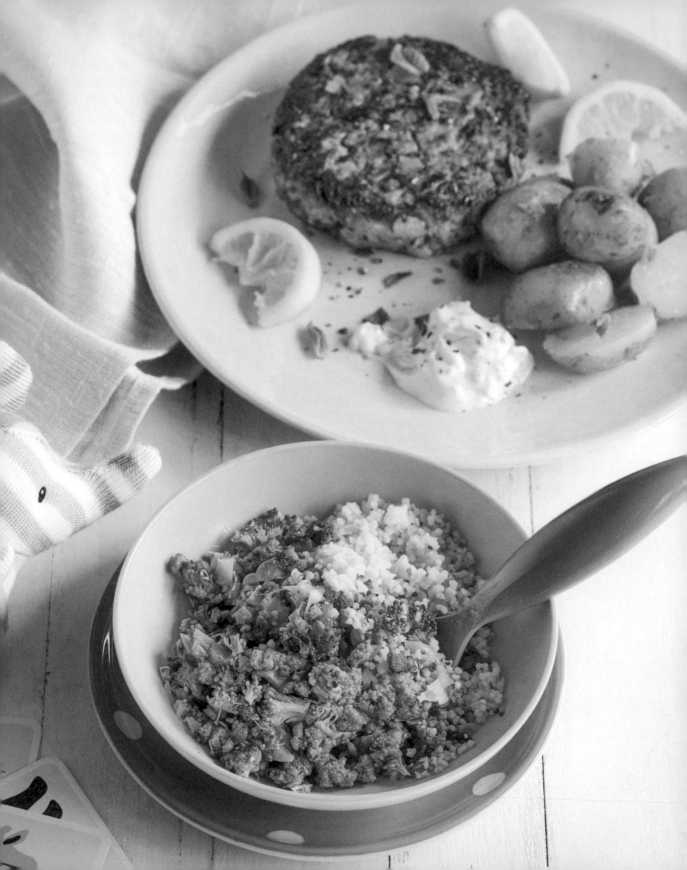

BABY PORK WITH APPLE & BROCCOLI

YOU PORK & APPLE BURGERS WITH TZATZIKI

Although there are concerns around some of the bugs it can contain, so long as you store and cook it correctly pork is considered safe to offer to babies. It is a good source of easily absorbed iron as well as other important B vitamins and minerals such as zinc and magnesium. Please note: only give your baby fresh pork, not cured or smoked pork products such as ham or bacon, since they contain high levels of salt.

Preparation time: 10 mins
Cooking time: 20 mins

TO PREPARE

250g pork mince

2 spring onions

6 cubes frozen apple purée, thawed, or 6 tbsp (90ml) fresh apple purée

FOR BABY

A drizzle of olive oil

2 tbsp (30ml) of the pork mixture

A handful of chopped broccoli florets

25g couscous

3 tbsp (45ml) boiling water

FOR YOU

Serves 2

4 wholegrain crackers

The remaining pork mixture

2 tsp (10ml) wholegrain mustard

A handful of parsley leaves

1 egg

Tzatziki, to serve (see right)

Cooked new potatoes, to serve (optional)

Put the pork mince in a bowl. Use scissors to finely chop in the spring onions, then stir in the apple purée.

FOR BABY PORK WITH APPLE & BROCCOLI

Heat the oil in a pan, add the pork mixture and chopped broccoli florets and cook gently for 6–8 minutes.

Meanwhile, place the couscous in a bowl and add the boiling water. Cover and leave to stand for 5 minutes, then fluff with a fork to separate the grains. Stir in the pork mixture.

FOR YOU PORK & APPLE BURGERS WITH TZATZIKI

Preheat the grill to medium-hot. Put the crackers in a food bag and crush with a rolling pin.

Place the pork mixture in a bowl, then stir in the crushed crackers, mustard, parsley leaves and egg. Use your hands to mix the ingredients until well combined, then shape into two burgers.

Grill the burgers in a foil-lined tray for 18–20 minutes, turning once, until golden and completely cooked through.

Serve with the tzatziki. Add cooked new potatoes to make a more substantial meal.

PERFECT TZATZIKI

To make tzatziki, put about 4 tbsp (60ml) plain Greek yogurt in a bowl. Peel ¼ cucumber, then cut in half lengthways and scoop out the seeds with a teaspoon. Finely dice or grate the remaining cucumber and put it on some kitchen paper. Squeeze to remove as much liquid as possible, then add the cucumber to the yogurt with a pinch of salt and ground black pepper, 1 crushed peeled garlic clove and a squeeze of lemon juice. You could also add some chopped herbs, such as dill or mint, if you have them.

BABY MINCED LAMB WITH ROOT MASH

YOU LAMB FILO PARCELS

Good-quality lamb contains valuable amounts of healthy fats and is an excellent source of vitamin B_{12} and a very good source of protein, selenium, and niacin. It is also a good source of zinc and phosphorus. If you are short on time, then rather than make folded parcels with the filo pastry, you can make twists. Follow the same method, but rather than fold, gather all the ends together and twist firmly once.

**Preparation time: 10 mins,
plus extra 10 mins for filo parcels
Cooking time 25 mins,
plus extra 10-12 mins for filo parcels**

TO PREPARE
A drizzle of olive oil

2 spring onions

250g minced lamb

3 carrots

2 parsnips

A pat of butter

1 tbsp (15ml) crème fraîche

FOR BABY
2 tbsp (30ml) of the lamb mixture

2 tbsp (30ml) of the mash

FOR YOU
Serves 2

2 tbsp (30ml) butter

The remaining lamb mixture

The remaining mash

1 tsp (5ml) ground cinnamon

1 tsp (5ml) ground cumin

1 tbsp (15ml) pine nuts

8 sheets of filo pastry

You can double the quantity of the lamb mixture to make extra parcels that you can freeze and keep for another day. Add other ingredients such as currants, pistachios, walnuts or cranberries to jazz them up.

Heat a drizzle of olive oil in a pan. Use scissors to chop in the spring onions, then cook for 2–3 minutes, until softened. Add the minced lamb and cook for a further 8 minutes, until cooked through.

Peel and chop the carrots and parsnips, put in a pan of boiling water and cook for 10 minutes, until soft. Alternatively, cook the diced vegetables with a drop of water in a covered bowl in the microwave on High for about 4 minutes, until tender, checking them halfway through.

Drain the cooked carrot and parsnip and place in a food processor with the butter and crème fraîche and whizz to make a smooth mash.

FOR BABY MINCED LAMB WITH ROOT MASH
Simply put the lamb mixture and the mash in a pan, stir to combine, and heat through.

FOR YOU LAMB FILO PARCELS
Preheat the oven to 200ºC (Gas 6). Melt the butter in a small pan or in the microwave.

Mix the lamb and mash together in a bowl and stir in the spices and pine nuts.

Take one sheet of filo, brush it with melted butter, then top this with another layer of filo. Keep the rest under a tea towel or cling film to prevent it from drying out while you work. Cut the two-layer filo into two long strips and stack these up so you have a four-layer strip.

Place a spoonful of the filling mixture at the thin end of the pastry nearest you. Fold a corner of the dough across to form a triangle. Brush with a little melted butter and fold upwards. Continue folding, across then up until you reach the end of the pastry. Repeat with the rest of the filo and filling until you have four triangular parcels.

Brush with a little more butter, place on a baking sheet and bake for 10–12 minutes, until crisp and golden.

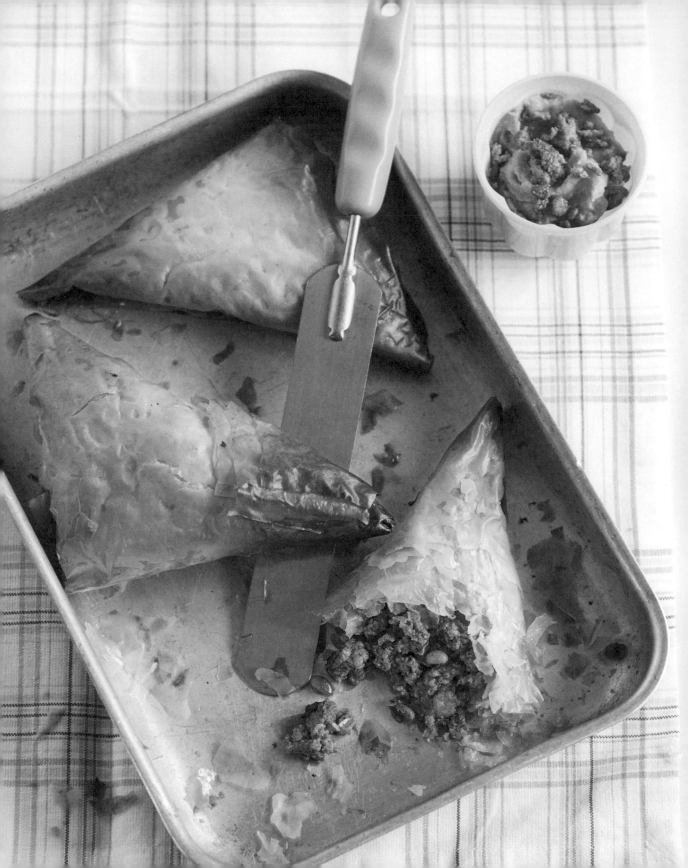

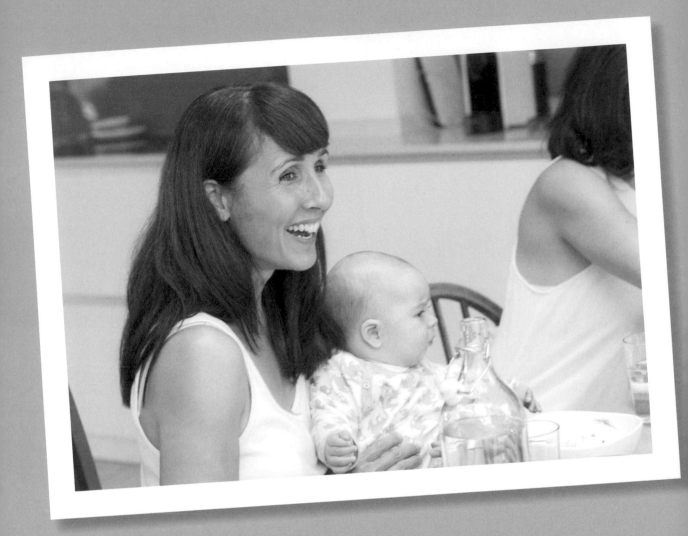
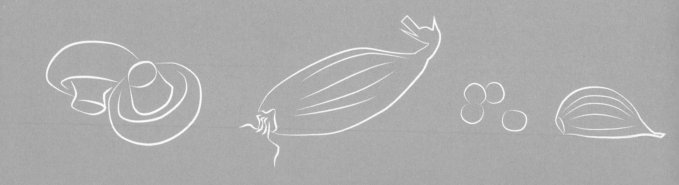

STAGE 3
FAMILY MEALS

Eating together is good for the whole family, it will help your baby develop healthy eating habits and build a healthy relationship with food and it provides the perfect opportunity for the rest of the family to eat more nutritiously. I truly believe it is worth the effort, even if you only manage it a few times a week. Once the TV is off and all other distractions are put to one side, there are not many things more enjoyable than sharing home cooked food while you chat and relax. The food doesn't have to be gourmet, just think Mediterranean-style, lots of food plonked in the middle of the table for everyone to help themselves. When scientists have looked into the subject, their research has proved the benefits by showing that children who eat 5-6 meals a week with their family are more likely to do better at school and less likely to engage in anti-social behaviours. Family meals provide a chance for your baby to learn the mechanics of eating, and the social skills of being together around the table, plus they also provide the chance to bond fostering warmth, security and feelings of belonging.

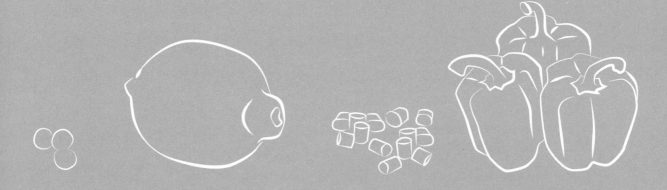

ROAST VEG ORZO

Orzo is pasta that looks more like large grains of rice, so is perfect for your baby and can be enjoyed by everyone without the need for special baby pasta. It goes well with this lovely ratatouille-style sauce, which you can beef up with some leftover cooked chicken if you have some.

Preparation time: 15 mins
Cooking time: 45-55 mins
Serves 4 and your baby

INGREDIENTS
2 tbsp (30ml) olive oil

2 aubergines, diced

3 courgettes, diced

3 red or yellow peppers, deseeded and diced

2 red onions, peeled and diced

4 garlic cloves, peeled and crushed

A handful of fresh basil, stalks chopped and leaves torn

6 ripe tomatoes, diced

400g canned chopped tomatoes

1 tbsp (15ml) balsamic vinegar

300g orzo

ADDITIONAL INGREDIENTS
A handful of basil leaves

Grated rind of ½ lemon

A pinch of salt and ground black pepper

Crusty fresh bread and a green salad, to serve

Heat the oil in a large pan over a medium heat. Add the aubergines, courgettes and peppers and fry for around 5 minutes, until golden and softened, but not cooked through. Spoon the vegetables into a large bowl.

Add the onion, garlic and basil stalks to the pan with another drizzle of oil, if needed. Fry for 10–15 minutes, or until softened and golden.

Return the cooked aubergine, courgettes and peppers to the pan and stir in the fresh and canned tomatoes and the balsamic vinegar. Fill the empty tomato can with water and add this to the pan, then stir in the orzo.

Mix well, breaking up the tomatoes with the back of a spoon. Cover the pan and simmer, uncovered, over a low heat for 30–35 minutes.

FOR BABY Serve your baby's portion and gently crush the chunkier pieces of vegetable, if necessary.

FOR EVERYBODY ELSE Tear in the basil leaves, add the lemon zest and season with a pinch of salt and ground black pepper. Serve with some crusty fresh bread and a green salad.

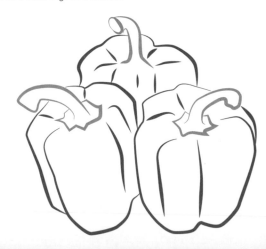

EDAMAME RISOTTO

Risotto takes a little bit of time to make, but it's extremely versatile – you can throw any veg or leftover meats into it. Risotto rice has a higher GI than most other rice types, but you can counter this by adding plenty of high-fibre, high-protein ingredients such as soybeans.

Preparation time: 10 mins
Cooking time: 30 mins
Serves 4 and your baby

INGREDIENTS
1 litre hot low-salt vegetable stock

2 tbsp (30ml) rapeseed oil

1 onion, peeled and finely diced

300g risotto rice

200g frozen soybeans, defrosted

ADDITIONAL INGREDIENTS
2 tbsp (30ml) ricotta

200g green beans, trimmed and steamed for 7–8 minutes, until tender

100g soft goat's cheese

Keep the stock warm in a pan over a low heat while you prepare the rest of the risotto.

Heat the oil in a large pan over a medium heat. Add the onion and cook gently for 10 minutes, until it turns soft and translucent.

Increase the heat a little and stir in the risotto rice, making sure each grain is coated in the oil. Cook the rice for 1–2 minutes, until the grains become translucent.

Add a ladleful of stock to the rice, reduce the heat and stir through. Once the stock is absorbed, add another ladleful and keep adding the stock, a ladleful at a time, waiting for stock to be absorbed before adding more. Stir continuously for about 18–20 minutes, until all of the stock has been absorbed and the rice is tender.

Add the soybeans to the risotto. Increase the heat and stir for a few minutes to heat everything through.

FOR BABY Remove 2–3 tbsp (30–45ml) for your baby and stir through the ricotta. Give your baby a couple of the steamed green beans.

FOR EVERYBODY ELSE Slice the remaining steamed green beans into small pieces and stir into the risotto with half of the goat's cheese. Just before serving, dot the risotto with the leftover goat's cheese.

MUSHROOM QUINOA RISOTTO

Quinoa and risotto rice blend nicely together to give a nutty flavour to the mushrooms.
Also, because the quinoa has a higher protein and fibre content than risotto rice,
the GI is lower, providing longer-lasting satisfaction.

Preparation time: 20 mins
Cooking time: 30 mins
Serves 4 and your baby

INGREDIENTS

15g mixed dried mushrooms

300ml boiling water

900ml low-salt chicken or vegetable stock

2 tbsp (30ml) olive oil

400g mushrooms (such as white, chestnut or a mixture), wiped clean and sliced

1 onion, peeled and chopped

2 garlic cloves, peeled and crushed

175g dried quinoa

175g risotto rice

100ml apple juice

2 tbsp (30ml) grated Parmesan cheese

A handful of chives, snipped

Spinach and pine nut salad, to serve

SPINACH AND PINE NUT SALAD

200g baby spinach leaves

½ cucumber, diced

5 sun-dried tomatoes in oil, drained and roughly chopped

1 tbsp (15ml) balsamic vinegar

Juice of ½ lemon

4 tbsp (60ml) pine nuts

Place the dried mushrooms in a bowl, cover with the boiling water and leave to soak for 10 minutes. Drain, reserving the liquid, then chop the mushrooms.

Put the stock in a large pan, add the dried mushroom liquid and slowly bring to the boil. Leave on a gentle simmer.

Heat half the oil in a large pan, add the sliced mushrooms and sauté over a high heat for 2–3 minutes, until golden brown. Transfer to a plate and set aside.

Add the remaining oil to the pan, add the onion and sauté for about 10 minutes, until softened. Add the chopped rehydrated mushrooms, garlic, quinoa and rice and stir for 30 seconds to coat the grains with the oil.

Add the apple juice and gently simmer, stirring, until the liquid has evaporated. Add a ladleful of the hot stock to the rice mixture and cook, stirring until the liquid has been absorbed. Repeat this process for about 20 minutes, until the rice is tender and the stock has all been used. Stir in the reserved mushrooms, Parmesan and chives.

FOR BABY Transfer 2 tbsp (30ml) to a bowl and serve.

FOR EVERYBODY ELSE Serve with the spinach and pine nut salad.

SPINACH AND PINE NUT SALAD
Place the spinach in a bowl with the cucumber and tomatoes, drizzle over the vinegar and lemon juice and scatter over the pine nuts.

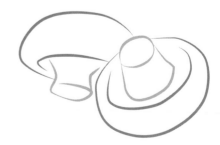

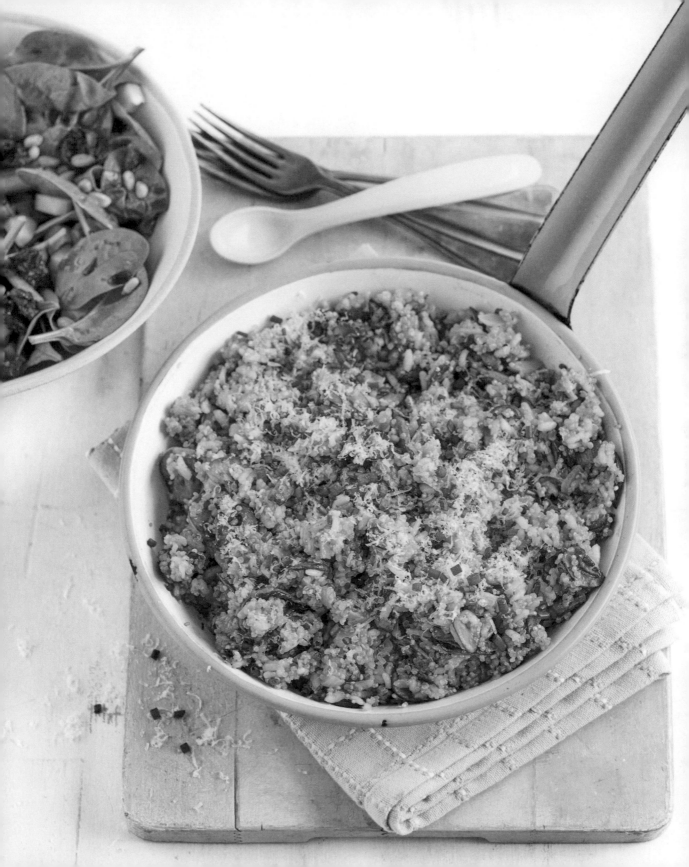

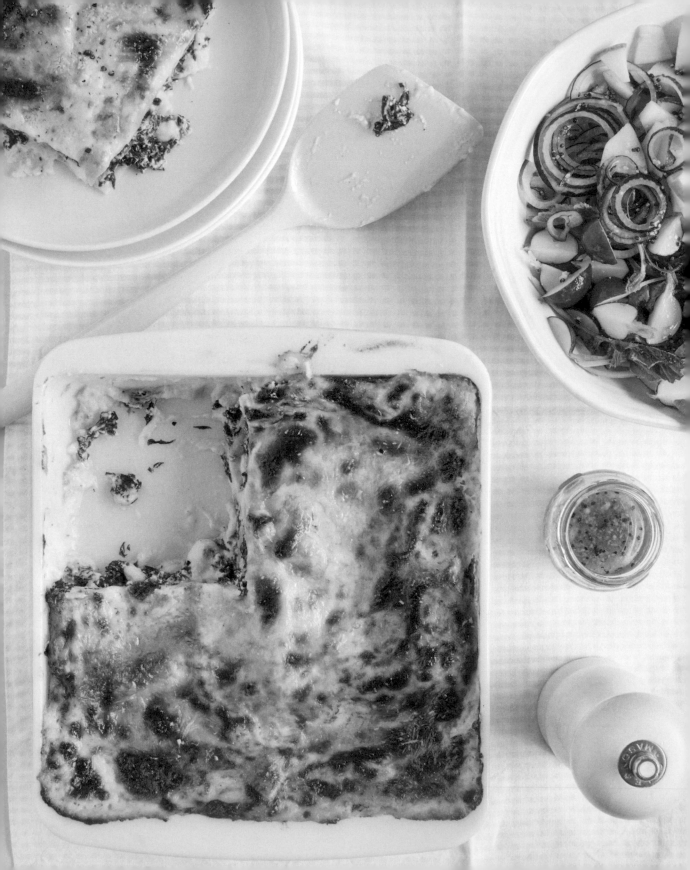

SPINACH & RICOTTA LASAGNE

This is a cheesy, creamy lasagne that everyone will love. It usually contains cashew nuts stirred into the spinach and ricotta mixture, but since whole nuts are not suitable for a baby these have been omitted. However, if you like, you can serve a handful on the side or add some to the radish salad.

Preparation time: 20 mins
Cooking time: 30-40 mins
Serves 4 and your baby

INGREDIENTS
50g butter

50g plain flour

850ml milk

1 bay leaf

100g Cheddar cheese, grated

100g mozzarella cheese, grated

600g spinach

225g ricotta

150ml crème fraîche

½ tsp (2.5ml) grated nutmeg

Ground black pepper

12 oven-ready lasagne sheets

3 tbsp (45ml) Parmesan cheese

Radish, fennel and apple salad, to serve

RADISH, FENNEL & APPLE SALAD
1 tsp (5ml) grain mustard

1 garlic clove, crushed

1 tbsp (15ml) cider vinegar

Juice from ½ lemon

2 tbsp (30ml) olive oil

10 radishes, trimmed and quartered

1 fennel bulb, trimmed and finely sliced

½ red onion, peeled and finely sliced

2 apples, cored and finely sliced

A handful of mint leaves, torn

Preheat the oven to 180°C (Gas 4). Melt the butter in a pan, add the flour and cook for 30 seconds. Gradually stir in the milk, add the bay leaf and heat gently, whisking or stirring continuously, until it thickens to make a smooth sauce.

Turn down the heat to its lowest setting and allow the sauce to cook gently for 5 minutes. Stir in the Cheddar and mozzarella, then remove the pan from the heat and discard the bay leaf.

Remove the stalks from the spinach, then wash the leaves thoroughly in cold water and shake them dry. Put the spinach leaves in a large pan, cover and place over a medium heat for about 2 minutes so they wilt.

Drain the spinach, and when it's cool enough to handle, squeeze it in your hands to get rid of the excess liquid, then chop it finely. Put it into a bowl, add the ricotta, crème fraîche and nutmeg and season with ground black pepper.

Assemble the lasagne by spreading one-quarter of the cheese sauce into the bottom of a lasagne dish (approximately 35 x 25cm), then one-third of the spinach mixture, followed by four lasagne sheets. Repeat the whole process, finishing with a layer of pasta, the rest of the sauce and the Parmesan sprinkled on top.

Bake for 50–60 minutes, until the top is golden and bubbling.

FOR BABY Transfer a portion to a bowl and chop it into small pieces.

FOR EVERYBODY ELSE Serve with radish, fennel and apple salad.

RADISH, FENNEL & APPLE SALAD
Put the mustard, garlic, vinegar, lemon juice and oil into a bowl and whisk to make a dressing.

Assemble the radishes, fennel, onion and apple on a platter and drizzle over the dressing. Scatter over the mint leaves.

CHEESY CHICKPEA GRATIN

Here's a healthier alternative to macaroni cheese that is higher in both fibre and protein but is just as creamy and comforting. The bacon is too high in salt to give to your baby but will add extra flavour for you. If you wanted to keep the dish veggie, substitute the bacon for slices of grilled mushrooms.

Preparation time: 15 mins
Cooking time: 30 mins
Serves 4 and your baby

INGREDIENTS
4 slices of wholemeal bread

450g spinach

2 tbsp (30ml) olive oil

4 red onions, peeled and roughly chopped

2 garlic cloves, peeled and finely sliced

1 tbsp (15ml) plain flour

400g canned chickpeas, drained

300ml low-salt vegetable stock

300g crème fraîche

100g Cheddar cheese, grated

ADDITIONAL INGREDIENTS
4 bacon rashers

4 large tomatoes, sliced

50g Parmesan cheese, grated

Preheat the oven to 180°C (Gas 4). Place the bread slices into a food processor and whizz until you have breadcrumbs.

Wash the spinach and place in a pan with just the water clinging to its leaves. Cover and steam for 2–3 minutes, until the leaves have wilted. Drain, squeeze out the excess water and finely chop.

Heat the oil in a large pan over a medium heat and add the onion and garlic. Cook gently for 10 minutes, until the onion is soft and translucent, then stir in the flour. Add the chickpeas, stock and crème fraîche to the pan and stir to warm through.

Add the spinach and cook for 1 minute before transferring to a large ovenproof dish. Sprinkle over the breadcrumbs and cheese and bake in the oven for 30 minutes, until the top is golden and crunchy.

FOR BABY Remove their portion and mash gently with a fork.

FOR EVERYBODY ELSE While the gratin is baking, preheat the grill to its highest setting. Place the bacon on a baking sheet. Cut the tomatoes into thick slices and place next to the bacon. Grill for 2–3 minutes, then turn over the bacon and tomatoes and sprinkle the Parmesan on the tomato slices. Return to the grill for another 2 minutes. Serve alongside the gratin.

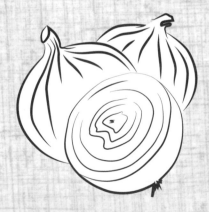

FRITTATA

Frittata makes a lovely light supper, ready in minutes and versatile for using up any leftover veg. The natural sweetness of the sweet potato and roasted red peppers make this a great choice for your baby, but you can add sharper flavours with different veg or stronger cheeses if they are more tolerant of those flavours.

Preparation time: 10 mins
Cooking time: 10 mins
Serves 2 and your baby

INGREDIENTS

1 sweet potato, peeled and chopped

A drizzle of olive oil

1 spring onion, finely sliced

200g roasted red peppers from a jar, drained and finely chopped

6 eggs

2 tbsp (30ml) Cheddar, grated

A handful of chives, snipped

ADDITIONAL INGREDIENTS

6 ripe tomatoes, sliced or roughly chopped

A drizzle of balsamic vinegar

A drizzle of olive oil

Place the sweet potato in a pan of boiling water and cook for 8 minutes, until tender. Drain and set aside. Preheat the grill to high.

Heat the oil in a large frying pan, add the spring onion and pepper and cook for 2 minutes. Add the sweet potato and gently crush together.

Crack the eggs into a bowl and beat together, then add the chives and cheese and stir to combine. Pour the egg mixture into the pan and lower the heat. Cook for about 7–8 minutes, until the top has almost set. Pop under the grill for 2–3 minutes, until firm and golden.

FOR BABY Cut a slice for your baby and gently mash it if necessary. If your baby is older and can cope with finger foods, cut it into small pieces.

FOR EVERYBODY ELSE Combine the tomatoes, balsamic vinegar and olive oil, then serve with the remaining frittata.

CHOWDER

Chowder is a great option for your baby in terms of consistency as it is thicker than a soup but runnier than a stew. Give your baby a spoon and he will enjoy trying to feed himself. You can also give him some toasted soldiers, which he will love to dip in.

Preparation time: 15 mins
Cooking time: 20 mins
Serves 2 and your baby

INGREDIENTS

1 tbsp (15ml) olive oil

2 baby leeks, finely sliced

400g potatoes, peeled and cut into small cubes

1 litre low-salt fish stock

Grated rind of 1 lemon

300ml crème fraîche

330g no added salt or sugar canned corn, rinsed and drained

250g skinless and boneless salmon fillet, cut into chunks

250g skinless and boneless sustainable white fish fillet, cut into chunks

A handful of chives, snipped

A pinch of salt and ground black pepper

Granary bread, to serve (not to the baby)

Heat the oil in a large pan over a medium heat, add the leeks and fry gently for 5 minutes, until softened. Add the potatoes and cook for a further 1 minute. Add the stock and lemon zest, cover and simmer for 15 minutes, until the potatoes are tender.

Using a slotted spoon, remove half the potatoes and leeks from the stock and set aside.

Transfer the remaining potatoes, leeks and stock to a blender or food processor and whizz until smooth, then stir in the crème fraîche.

Return to the pan and add the corn and fish and cook for 5 minutes until the fish is cooked though and flakes easily.

FOR BABY Remove your baby's portion and gently mash the fish.

FOR EVERYBODY ELSE Add the reserved potatoes and leeks. Cook for another 1 minute, then stir in the chives and season with a pinch of salt and ground black pepper. Serve with a chunk of granary bread.

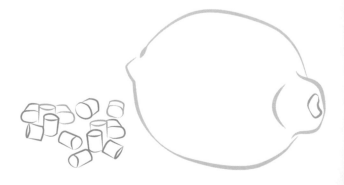

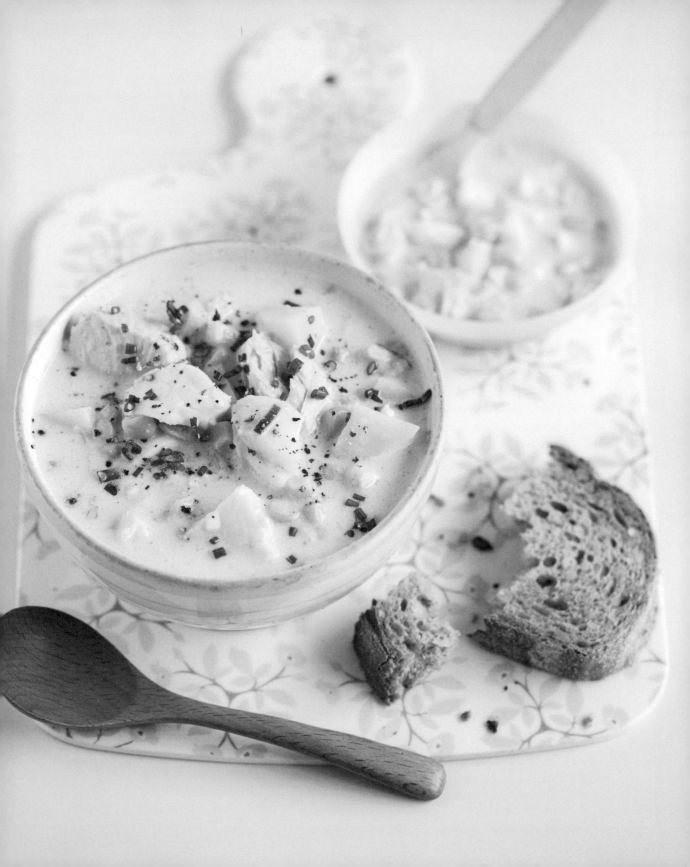

FISH CRUMBLE

Fish pie with a mashed potato topping is a great option for a nutritious family meal, but for a little twist, try this crumble topping instead. It adds crunch and extra fibre and has a lower GI than standard mash. As shellfish such as prawns and scallops can pose a slight risk of food poisoning, it is best to wait until your baby's immune system is better developed before offering them. The risks are minimal when good hygienic practice of handling, storing and cooking is observed.

Preparation time: 20 mins
Cooking time: 50-60 mins
Serves 4 and your baby

INGREDIENTS

3 eggs

1 tbsp (15ml) rapeseed oil

1 onion, peeled and chopped

1 bay leaf

50g flour

150ml apple juice

200ml milk

600g skinless and boneless fish fillet, cut into 3cm cubes, or ready mixed fish pie mix that doesn't include any shellfish

2 tbsp (30ml) chopped fresh dill

100g butter

150g wholemeal flour

150g oatmeal

50g Parmesan cheese, finely grated

A small bunch of flat leaf parsley, finely chopped

Steamed vegetables, to serve

ADDITIONAL INGREDIENTS

A drizzle of olive oil

200g raw tiger prawns

200g scallops

Preheat the oven to 200°C (Gas 6). Place the eggs in a pan of cold water, bring to the boil and simmer for 8 minutes, until hard-boiled. Drain and refill the pan with cold water. Keep the eggs in the water until they are just warm, then peel off the shells and finely chop the eggs.

Heat the oil in a large pan over a medium heat and gently sauté the onion with the bay leaf for about 10 minutes, until the onion is softened but not coloured.

Stir in the flour and cook for about 30 seconds before gradually adding the apple juice, stirring to prevent any lumps forming.

Add the milk in the same way, then bring to a simmer and cook for a few minutes until you have a thick sauce.

Gently stir in the fish and cook for a few minutes, then add the eggs and dill. Spoon the fish mixture into a large ovenproof dish and set aside.

To make the crumble topping, melt the butter in a large pan, then remove from the heat and stir in the flour, oatmeal, Parmesan and chopped parsley. Add a little oil if the mixture seems too dry.

Scatter the topping over the fish and cook in the preheated oven for 30–40 minutes, until the topping is golden and the filling is bubbling at the edges. It is a good idea to place the dish on a baking tray to catch any spills.

FOR YOUR BABY Remove their portion and serve with some steamed vegetables.

FOR EVERYBODY ELSE When the crumble is nearly ready, heat a drizzle of olive oil in a pan, add the prawns and scallops and cook for 2–3 minutes on each side until the prawns are pink and the scallops are just cooked through. Serve with the crumble and some steamed vegetables.

SALMON FISHCAKES

These fishcakes are a great way of getting easy and affordable salmon into your family's diet and everyone will love them, including your baby. The sweet potato gives them a slightly sweeter flavour than white potatoes would, which your baby may prefer. Sweet potatoes get their vibrant orange colour as they are a rich source of beta carotene which is needed for healthy skin and to boost immunity.

Preparation time: 15 min
Cooking time: 30 mins
Makes 5 fishcakes (1 for your baby)

INGREDIENTS
2 sweet potatoes, peeled and diced

6 multigrain crackers

2 cans (approximately 215g) red salmon in spring water, drained and flaked

4 spring onions, chopped

1 tbsp (15ml) chives, snipped

1 tbsp (15ml) dill, snipped

3 tbsp (45ml) plain flour

1 egg, beaten

Steamed green vegetables, such as sugar snap peas or mangetout, to serve (for baby)

CAPER, LETTUCE AND PEAS
200g frozen peas

A pat of butter

1 shallot, peeled and diced

1 garlic clove, peeled and crushed

A handful of thyme leaves

2 tbsp (30ml) capers

½ iceberg lettuce, shredded

A pinch of salt and ground black pepper

A handful of fresh mint

Preheat the oven to 200ºC (Gas 6).

Put the potatoes in a pan of boiling water and cook for 8–10 minutes, until tender, then drain and leave to cool and for the steam to evaporate in a sieve.

Meanwhile, place the crackers in a food bag and crush with a rolling pin.

Transfer the potatoes to a bowl and add the salmon, spring onions and herbs and mix well.

Place the flour, egg and crushed crackers on to three plates. Divide the fish mixture into five portions and mould each into a fish cake (make one portion smaller than the others, for your baby). Dip each fish cake carefully first into the flour, then the egg, then the crushed crackers.

Place on a baking sheet and bake for 20 minutes, until golden.

FOR YOUR BABY Gently mash your baby's fish cake and serve with some steamed sugar snap peas or mangetout for her to hold.

FOR EVERYBODY ELSE Serve with capers, lettuce and peas.

CAPER, LETTUCE AND PEAS
Put the peas in a pan of boiling water and cook for 5 minutes. Drain and set aside.

Heat the butter in the pan, add the shallot, garlic and thyme leaves and cook for 5 minutes, until softened.

Add the capers, peas and lettuce, season with a pinch of salt and ground black pepper and cook for a few more minutes, until the lettuce wilts. Stir in the mint.

FISH STEW

This is a light, tasty stew that is simple to make and ready in minutes. You can use frozen white fish if you don't have the fresh type. Fennel has a strong aniseed flavour that your baby may not be too keen on so you might want to leave it out from his portion. However, there is no reason you can't offer it – he'll soon let you know whether he likes it or not!

Preparation time: 10 mins
Cooking time: 20 mins
Serves 2 and your baby

INGREDIENTS
A drizzle of olive oil

1 shallot, peeled and finely chopped

1 garlic clove, peeled and finely chopped

100g skinless white fish fillet

50g frozen peas

300ml low-salt vegetable stock

200g canned chopped tomatoes

200g couscous

300ml boiling water

A squeeze of lemon juice

ADDITIONAL INGREDIENTS
A drizzle of olive oil

1 fennel bulb, finely chopped

A splash of vermouth or dry white wine

250g mixed seafood

200g baby spinach leaves

A pinch of salt and ground black pepper

Heat the oil in a large pan, add the shallot and garlic and cook for 5 minutes, until softened. Add the fish, peas, stock and tomatoes. Bring to the boil and simmer for 15 minutes. The fish will break up.

While the sauce is simmering, place the couscous in a bowl, add the boiling water and the lemon juice, then stir, cover with cling film and allow to stand for 8–10 minutes.

FOR BABY Transfer 2 tbsp (30ml) of the couscous into a bowl, add 2 tbsp (30ml) of the fish stew and gently mix.

FOR EVERYBODY ELSE In another pan, heat a drizzle of olive oil, add the fennel and cook for 5 minutes, until soft. Add the vermouth or white wine and let it bubble for a minute, then stir in the seafood and spinach to heat through. Season with a pinch of salt and ground black pepper.

Tip the fennel and seafood mixture into the remaining stew and mix together. Serve with the couscous.

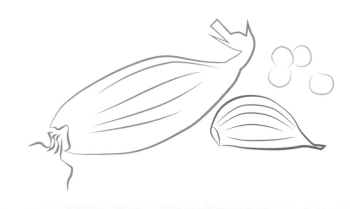

TROUT WITH CRUSHED PEAS

Here's a quick and easy supper if you want something on the table in less than 15 minutes. The trout counts towards your oily fish intake and is high in healthy omega-3 fats. The peas add protein, fibre and vitamin C. The peas add protein, vitamin C and a type of fibre that helps boost the number of friendly bacteria in the gut, reducing your risk of picking up infections.

Preparation time: 5 mins
Cooking time: 8 mins
Serves 2 and your baby

INGREDIENTS

2 x 150g trout fillets

A drizzle of olive oil

2 limes, 1 peeled and sliced into rounds and the other juiced

250g fresh or frozen peas

1 tbsp (15ml) butter

1 tbsp (15ml) crème fraîche

ADDITIONAL INGREDIENTS

A bunch of fresh coriander, finely chopped

Salt and ground black pepper

Preheat the oven to 180°C (Gas 4). Lay the trout fillets in an ovenproof dish and drizzle with olive oil. Place the slices of lime on the fish and roast in the oven for 8 minutes, until the fish is cooked through.

Meanwhile, cook the peas in boiling water for 3 minutes, until tender. Drain and place in a bowl. Add the butter, crème fraîche and lime juice and use a potato masher to crush the peas into a coarse mash.

Remove the fish from the oven and flake the flesh from the skin.

FOR BABY Transfer 2 tbsp (30ml) of the crushed peas to your baby's bowl and stir through some of the flaked fish.

FOR EVERYBODY ELSE Stir most of the fresh coriander through the remaining crushed peas and season with a pinch of salt and plenty of ground black pepper. Serve the remaining trout on top on the mashed peas and sprinkle with the rest of the coriander.

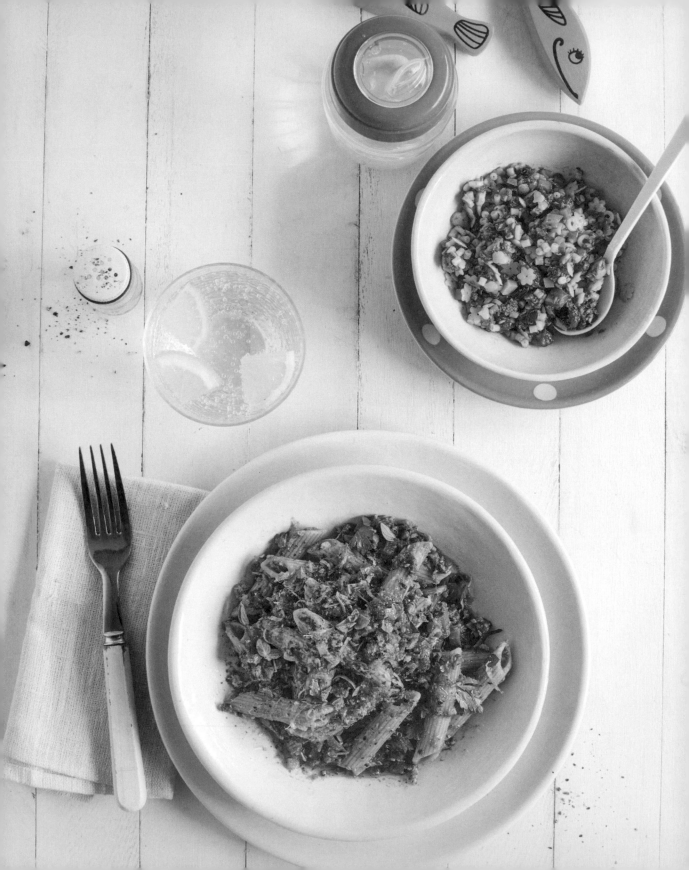

SARDINE BOLOGNAISE

Everyone loves spaghetti bolognaise and here is a clever twist using sardines instead of meat. It might sound a bit odd, but it really works as the fish breaks up to resemble soft mince and goes well with the Italian flavours. It's a great way for everyone to enjoy their recommended oily fish.

Preparation time 10 mins
Cooking time: 25 mins
Serves 4 and your baby

INGREDIENTS

1 tbsp (15ml) olive oil, plus extra for drizzling

1 onion, peeled and finely chopped

1 large carrot, peeled and finely chopped

1 celery stick, finely chopped

1 green pepper, deseeded and finely chopped

250g brown mushrooms, wiped clean and diced

4 x 120g cans of sardines, drained

400g canned chopped tomatoes

1 tbsp (15ml) tomato purée

1 tsp (5ml) dried Italian herbs

200g wholemeal pasta shapes

2 tbsp (30ml) baby pasta shapes (such as shells or letters)

ADDITIONAL INGREDIENTS

A drizzle of olive oil

4 slices of wholemeal bread

1 tbsp (15ml) flat leaf parsley, roughly chopped

1 tbsp (15ml) fresh oregano, roughly chopped

Grated rind of 1 lemon

1 tbsp (15ml) grated Parmesan cheese

Heat the oil in a large pan, add the onion and cook over a medium heat for about 10 minutes, until soft. Add the carrot, celery and green pepper and cook for 15 minutes. Add the mushrooms and cook for a further 5 minutes.

Stir in the sardines, chopped tomatoes, tomato purée and Italian herbs. Continue cooking gently for a further 5 minutes, during which time the sardines will break up.

Bring a large pan of water to the boil and cook the pasta according to the packet instructions. Cook your baby's pasta in a separate pan. Drain once cooked.

FOR BABY Place your baby's pasta in a bowl and stir through 2 tbsp (30ml) of the sardine bolognaise.

FOR EVERYBODY ELSE While the pasta is cooking, make a crunchy topping using the additional ingredients. Put the bread slices into a food processor and whizz until you have coarse breadcrumbs. Add the parsley, oregano, lemon rind and Parmesan and whizz again until everything is well combined and finely chopped.

Preheat the grill to its highest setting. Lightly grease the base and sides of an ovenproof dish with a little olive oil to prevent the pasta bake from sticking. Combine the pasta and sauce, then pour it into the dish and top with the breadcrumb mixture. Grill for 3–5 minutes, until the top is golden.

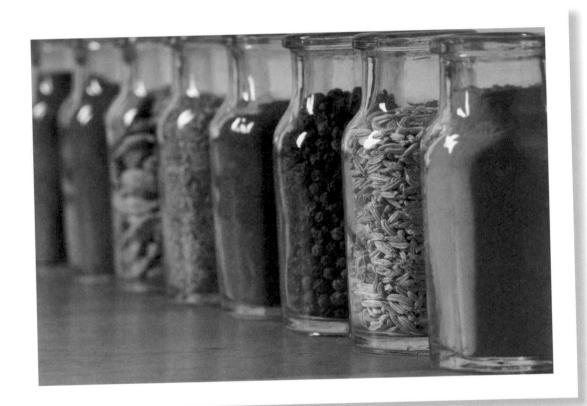

CHICKEN KORMA

You can introduce your baby to pungent spices including chilli early on. This will develop their enjoyment of a wide range of flavours and aromas and help to shape a healthy eating pattern as they get older. Build up the level of spiciness slowly; the merest hint will be enough the first time they try it. The spinach is a great way to add bulk without calories (just fibre and extra nutrients) and for no extra effort, but if you would like to add some to your baby's portion, then chop it finely before adding.

Preparation time: 15 mins
Cooking time: 20 mins
Serves 4 and your baby

INGREDIENTS

2 tbsp (30ml) rapeseed oil

2 large onions, peeled and chopped

A piece of fresh ginger, peeled and chopped

1 tsp (5ml) cumin seeds

2 tbsp (30ml) ground coriander

1 tbsp (15ml) ground cumin

½ tsp (2.5ml) chilli powder

2 garlic cloves, peeled and chopped

4 skinless chicken breasts, diced

1 bay leaf

Boiling water, to cover

120g ground almonds

4 tbsp (60ml) yogurt

Cooked brown basmati rice, to serve

ADDITIONAL INGREDIENTS

Extra chilli powder or chopped fresh chilli

A pinch of salt and ground black pepper

4 large handfuls of spinach leaves

3 tbsp (45ml) cashew nuts

A handful of fresh coriander leaves

Heat the oil in a large pan, add the onions and ginger and fry over a medium heat for 5 minutes, until softened.

Add the cumin seeds, ground coriander, ground cumin and chilli powder and fry for 1–2 minutes, until the spices release their aromas. Stir in the chopped garlic and fry for another minute.

Add the chicken pieces and bay leaf and allow the chicken to brown slightly over a medium heat. Pour in enough boiling water to just cover the chicken. Bring back to the boil, then reduce the heat to a simmer and cook gently for 15 minutes.

Stir the ground almonds into the yogurt, then add to the pan. Stir gently and continue cooking to allow the mixture to heat through.

FOR BABY Remove their portion and serve in a bowl with 1–2 tbsp (15–30ml) of the rice.

FOR EVERYBODY ELSE Add the extra chilli to your taste and season with a pinch of salt and ground black pepper. Add the spinach leaves and cook until they just wilt. Scatter over the cashew nuts and fresh coriander and serve with the rice.

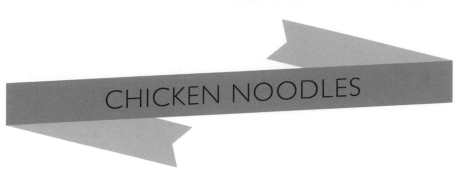

CHICKEN NOODLES

Your baby will love these soft, thick noodles and picking up the colourful pieces of pepper and carrot. The peanut butter adds a bit of stickiness so you can gently mash the noodles and chicken if you need a smoother texture. It also adds more protein and calcium. Add the peanuts, fresh chilli and soy sauce for everybody else to create a satisfying meal that is ready in minutes.

Preparation time, 10 mins
Cooking time: 15 mins
Serves 2 and your baby

INGREDIENTS
200g soba noodles

200g skinless chicken breast, cut into strips

1 tsp (15ml) Chinese five spice

1 tbsp (15ml) rapeseed oil

2 spring onions, chopped

1 carrot, cut into matchsticks

50g mangetout, finely sliced

1 red pepper, deseeded and finely sliced

2 tbsp (30ml) peanut butter

A splash of water

ADDITIONAL INGREDIENTS
2 tbsp (30ml) unsalted roasted peanuts

½ red chilli, deseeded and finely sliced (or a splash of chilli sauce)

A splash soy sauce

Cook the noodles in boiling water, according to the packet instructions. Drain well.

Place the chicken in a bowl, add the Chinese five spice and toss to coat the chicken. Heat the oil in a wok or large frying pan, add the chicken and cook for 10 minutes, until thoroughly cooked. Remove from the wok or pan and set aside.

Turn up the heat and allow the wok or pan to get very hot before adding the spring onions, carrot, mangetout and pepper. Stir-fry for 2–3 minutes.

Meanwhile, add the chicken to the wok or pan with the peanut butter. Add a splash of water and stir-fry for 2 minutes. Finally, add the noodles and cook for a further minute.

FOR BABY Remove your baby's portion and serve.

FOR EVERYBODY ELSE Add the remaining ingredients to the wok or pan and cook for 1–2 minutes.

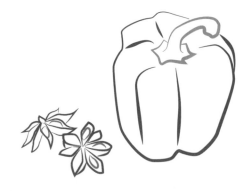

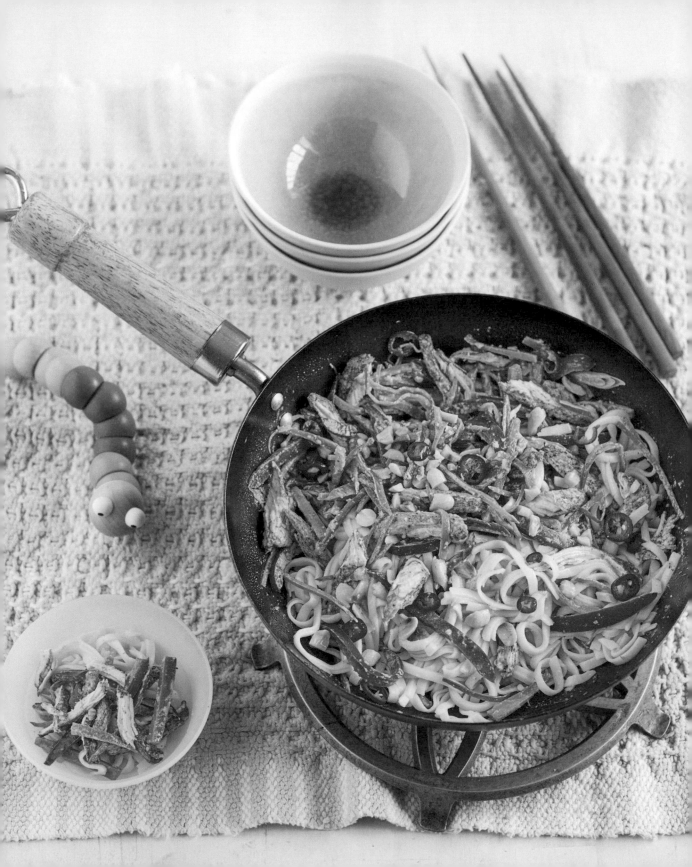

THAI TURKEY CURRY

Reserve a couple of the asparagus spears and steam or boil while the curry is cooking. Your baby will love holding and eating them while you're cooking. If the pieces of veg are too big, use a potato masher to mash the curry and rice together to make a smoother texture, but aim to get your baby used to lumpier pieces with each meal.

Preparation time 10 mins
Cooking time: 20 mins
Serves 2 and your baby

INGREDIENTS

1 tbsp (15ml) vegetable oil

2 tbsp (30ml) mild green curry paste

250g turkey mince

400ml canned coconut milk

Juice from 1 lime

1 tbsp (15ml) Thai fish sauce

50g green beans,
trimmed and finely sliced

100g asparagus spears,
trimmed and finely sliced

Basmati rice, to serve

1 tbsp (15ml) plain Greek yogurt

ADDITIONAL INGREDIENTS

50g baby corn

50g mangetout

A handful of fresh coriander leaves

Baby corn makes a good alternative to rice or noodles if you fancy a lower-carbohydrate option.

Heat the oil in a wok or large frying pan over a high heat until it is smoking. Add the green curry paste and stir-fry for 1–2 minutes, until fragrant.

Add the turkey mince and stir until coated in the curry paste. Continue to stir-fry for 1–2 minutes.

Add the coconut milk, lime juice and fish sauce and stir well. Bring to the boil, then reduce the heat until the mixture is simmering. Continue to simmer for 8–10 minutes, until the sauce has thickened.

Add the green beans and asparagus and continue to simmer for 2–3 minutes, stirring regularly, until tender.

FOR BABY Place 1–2 tbsp (15–30ml) basmati rice in a bowl and stir through 2 tbsp (30ml) of the turkey curry with 1 tbsp (15ml) plain Greek yogurt.

FOR EVERYBODY ELSE Add the baby corn and mangetout to the wok and cook for a further 2–3 minutes. Serve with the rice and sprinkle over the fresh coriander leaves.

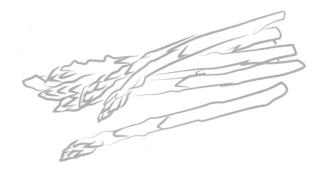

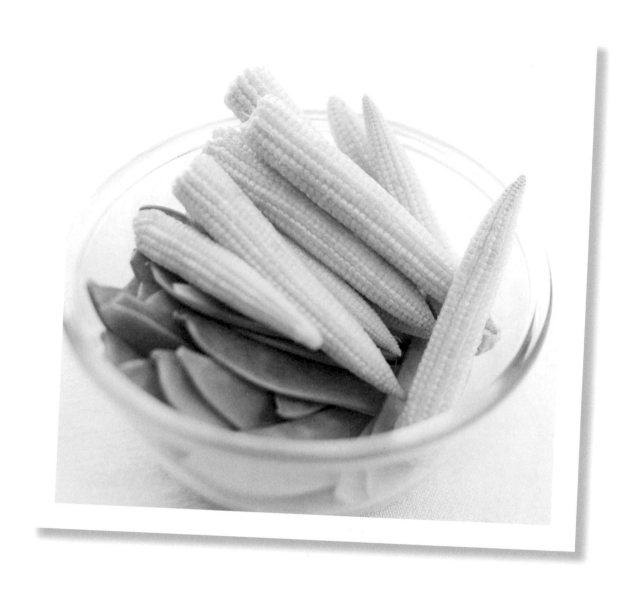

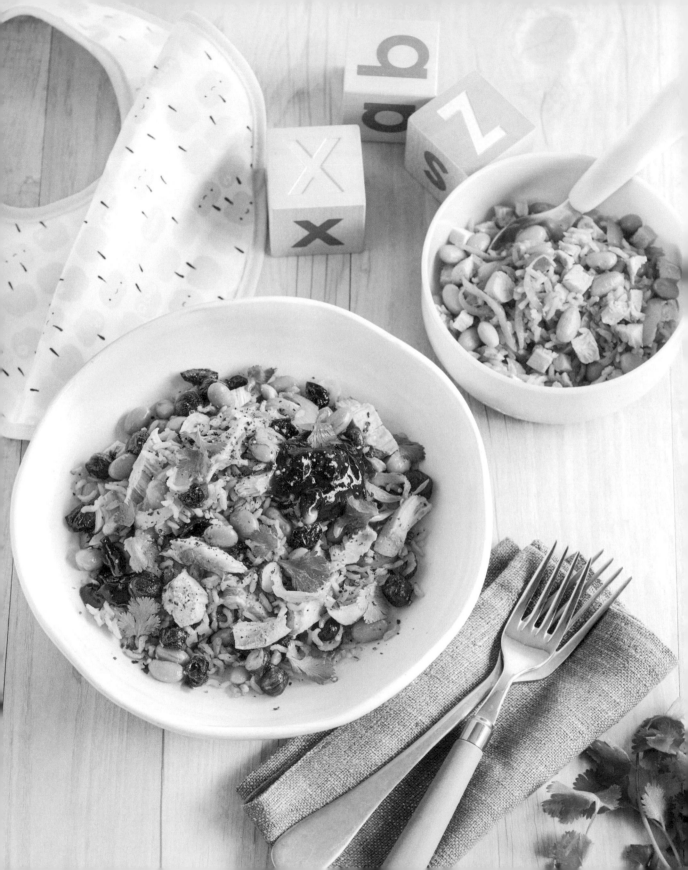

TURKEY PILAF

Pilaf is not sticky like risotto – the rice needs to be fluffy and light, so use good-quality basmati rice, which has a much lower GI than risotto rice. It you don't have leftover cooked turkey or chicken you can use a can of tuna, and frozen peas can replace the edamame beans. Stir through some whole hazelnuts and dried cranberries to add extra crunch and bite to everybody else's serving (not for the baby).

Preparation time: 10 mins
Cooking time: 30-35 mins
Serves 2 and your baby

INGREDIENTS
1 tbsp (15ml) olive oil

1 onion, peeled and chopped

1 garlic clove, peeled and crushed

4 cardamom pods, bashed

1 tsp (5ml) ground cumin

1 cinnamon stick

100g brown basmati rice

300ml low-salt vegetable stock

200g cooked turkey, shredded

100g frozen edamame

ADDITIONAL INGREDIENTS
30g whole hazelnuts

A pinch of salt and ground black pepper

1 tbsp (15ml) dried cranberries

A handful of fresh coriander, roughly chopped

A dollop of cranberry sauce

Heat the oil in a pan and gently fry the onion and garlic over a medium heat for about 10 minutes, until softened. Add the spices and rice and cook for 1–2 minutes.

Pour in the hot stock, reduce the heat to low and simmer, uncovered, for about 20–25 minutes or until the stock is nearly all absorbed.

Stir in the turkey and beans and continue to cook until everything is warmed through.

FOR BABY Serve your baby's portion in a bowl. The turkey might need to be chopped into smaller pieces.

FOR EVERYBODY ELSE Place a small frying pan over a medium heat and add the whole hazelnuts. Toast for a few minutes, stirring occasionally, until the nuts turn golden brown. Remove from the pan quickly as they will continue to cook in the pan and can burn easily.

Season the pilaf with a pinch of salt and ground black pepper, stir in the hazelnuts and cranberries and scatter over the fresh coriander. Divide between two bowls and serve with a dollop of cranberry sauce.

COOKING TURKEY FROM RAW

If you want to cook some turkey from raw, simply place 1 skinless turkey breast in a pan of simmering water and poach it for about 10 minutes, until cooked through.

SLOW-COOKED PORK WITH LENTILS

If you're thinking of entertaining some of your new baby friends (and their babies), here is a simple but sensational dish for everyone to share and enjoy. You can prepare it in minutes and then leave it to slowly cook all day while you get on with other things.

Preparation time, 10 mins
Cooking time: 4 hours
Serves 8 and your baby

INGREDIENTS

2kg pork shoulder on the bone

Olive oil, for greasing

200ml white wine vinegar

250ml apple juice or alcohol-free cider

3 onions, peeled and finely sliced

6 garlic cloves, peeled and sliced

200g dried Puy lentils, rinsed

Water

Steamed green beans,
to serve (for everybody)

Spicy refried beans and mustard, to serve
(for everybody apart from baby)

SPICY REFRIED BEANS

A drizzle of olive oil

2 onions, peeled and finely chopped

4 garlic cloves, peeled and finely chopped

1 tsp (5ml) chilli flakes

1 tbsp (15ml) cumin seeds

4 x 400g canned pinto beans,
rinsed and drained

2 tbsp (30ml) smoked paprika

A splash of water

A pinch of salt and ground black pepper

Preheat the oven to 170°C (Gas 3). Place the pork shoulder in a lightly oiled roasting tin. Pour over the vinegar and juice or cider, then scatter over the sliced onion and garlic.

Cover with parchment paper, then cover tightly in foil and cook in the preheated oven for 3 hours.

Remove the parchment paper and foil. Add the lentils to the roasting tin along with sufficient water to just cover the lentils, and return to the oven to cook for a further 1 hour.

Remove from the oven. The pork should be soft enough to shred easily.

FOR BABY Put some of the shredded pork and 2–3 tbsp (30–45ml) of the lentils in a bowl. Serve with a few steamed green beans.

FOR EVERYBODY ELSE Serve the pork with the spicy refried beans, some steamed green beans and plenty of mustard.

SPICY REFRIED BEANS

Heat the olive oil in a large frying pan, add the onion and garlic and cook over a medium heat for 8–10 minutes. Add the chilli flakes and cumin seeds and cook for a further minute.

Tip in the beans, paprika and a splash of water. Using a potato masher, break down the beans as they warm through, to make a rough purée. Season with a pinch of salt and ground black pepper.

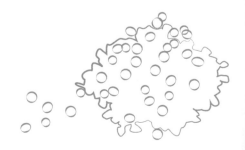

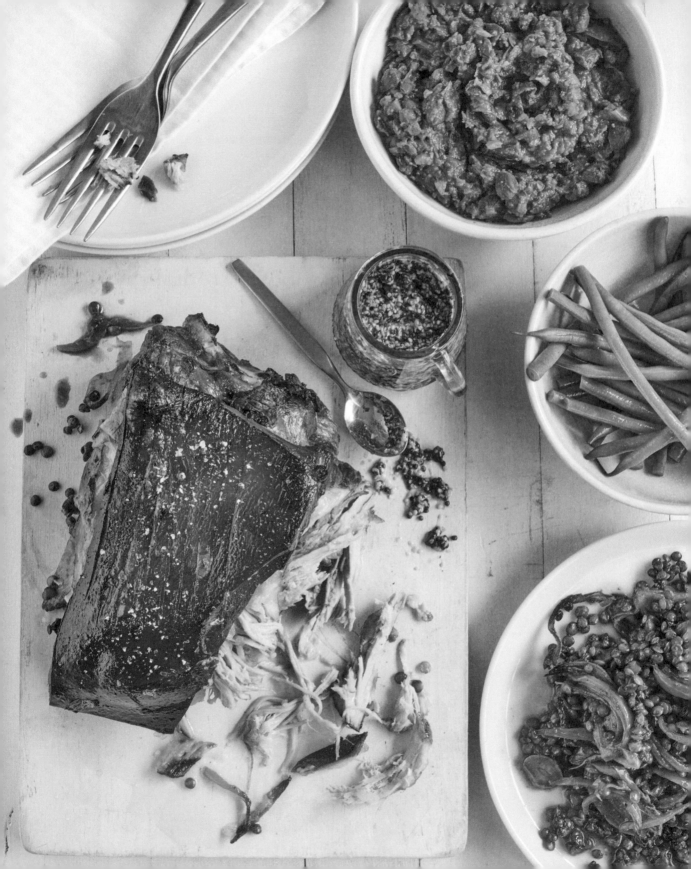

LAMB MEATBALLS

These meatballs are easy and versatile: you can make them with pork or turkey mince in exactly the same way, and the tomato sauce is rich and tasty yet so simple to make. Meats, such as lamb, pork and turkey are high in the amino acid, tryptophan, which is needed for the production of serotonin in the brain, often known as the feel-good hormone.

Preparation time: 20 mins
Cooking time: 20 mins
Serves 2 and your baby

INGREDIENTS

250g lamb mince (or pork or turkey)

1 red onion, peeled and chopped

1 small carrot, peeled and grated

1 tsp (5ml) fresh or dried oregano

1 egg, beaten

A drizzle of olive oil

1 garlic clove, peeled and chopped

400g canned chopped tomatoes

2 fresh tomatoes, roughly chopped

1 tbsp (15ml) tomato purée

200ml water

ADDITIONAL INGREDIENTS

200g kale

1 tsp (5ml) chilli flakes

1 tbsp (15ml) Worcestershire sauce

A pinch of salt and ground black pepper

A squeeze of lemon

Place the mince in a bowl with half of the onion, and the carrot, oregano and egg. Mix well and shape into 15 small meatballs. Use dampened hands to prevent the mixture sticking, if necessary.

Drizzle a little olive oil into a large pan and fry the meatballs over a medium heat for about 5 minutes until browned all over, then remove with a slotted spoon and set aside.

Drizzle a little more oil into the same pan and add the remaining onion and the garlic. Cook for about 10 minutes, until softened.

Add the canned and fresh tomatoes, tomato purée and water. Bring to the boil, then simmer, uncovered, for 3–4 minutes.

Add the meatballs, cover the pan and simmer for 20 minutes, stirring occasionally.

FOR BABY Remove your baby's portion and gently crush the meatballs into the sauce.

FOR EVERYBODY ELSE While the sauce is cooking, steam the kale. Stir the chilli flakes and Worcestershire sauce into the tomato sauce and season with a pinch of salt and plenty of ground black pepper. Squeeze some lemon juice over the kale and serve alongside the meatballs.

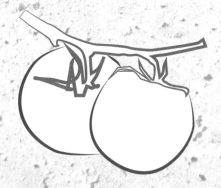

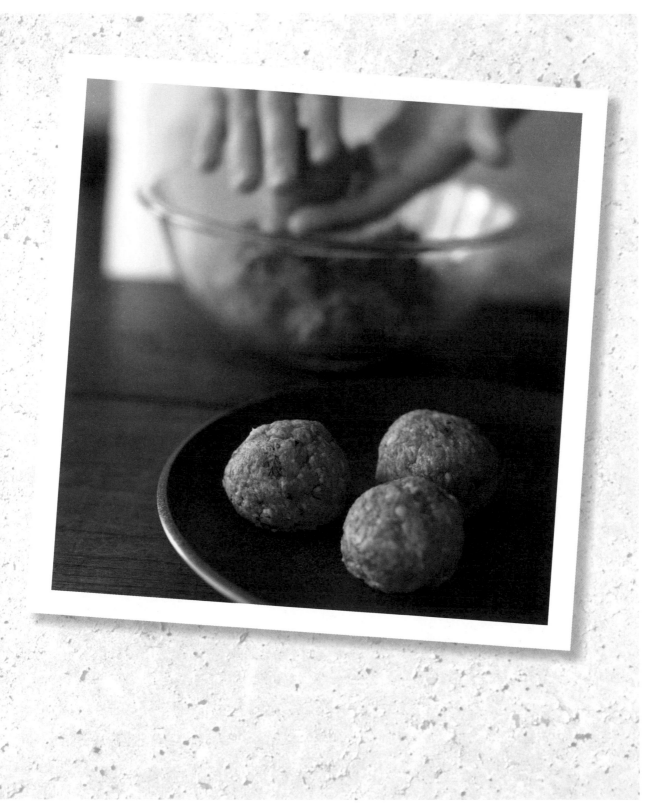

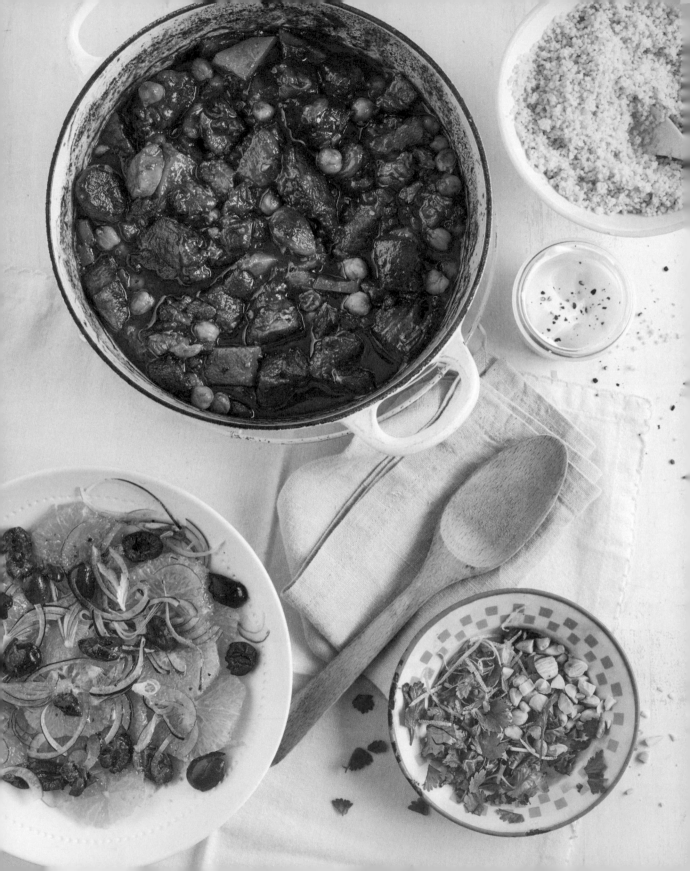

LAMB TAGINE

Preparation time: 20 mins
Cooking time: 90 mins
Serves 4 and your baby

INGREDIENTS

1 tbsp (15ml) olive oil

1 large onion, peeled and finely chopped

2 garlic cloves, peeled and finely chopped

1 tbsp (15ml) ras el hanout

400g lamb shoulder or neck, diced

200g butternut squash, peeled and diced

400g canned chickpeas, rinsed and drained

200g ready-to-eat dried apricots, chopped

400g canned chopped tomatoes

500ml low-salt beef stock

Couscous or brown basmati rice, to serve (for everybody)

Plain Greek yogurt, to serve (for baby)

Orange, red onion and black olive salad, to serve (for everybody apart from baby)

ADDITIONAL INGREDIENTS

A pinch of salt and ground black pepper

50g almonds

Grated rind of 1 lemon

A small bunch of fresh coriander, roughly chopped

ORANGE, RED ONION & BLACK OLIVE SALAD

2 large oranges

1 tbsp (15ml) olive oil

Juice of 1 lemon

1 tbsp (15ml) white wine vinegar

A pinch of salt and ground black pepper

½ red onion, peeled and sliced

2 tbsp (30ml) black olives, pitted and halved

Introduce your baby to delicious Moroccan flavours with this simple, tasty lamb tagine. Make it while your baby has her daytime sleep and then you can have it ready and waiting at that pressure point of the day when she is hungry and there may be other mouths to feed, too.

Preheat the oven to 180ºC (Gas 5). Heat the oil in a flameproof casserole, add the onion and cook for 10 minutes over a medium heat, until softened. Add the garlic and ras el hanout and cook, stirring, for a couple of minutes more.

Add the lamb, butternut squash, chickpeas and apricots to the casserole, then pour over the tomatoes and stock. Bring to the boil.

Put the lid on and transfer the casserole to the oven. After 1 hour, turn down the oven to 150ºC (Gas 2), stir the tagine and return to the oven, uncovered, for a further 30 minutes.

FOR BABY Serve your baby's portion in a bowl with 2 tbsp (30ml) rice or couscous. Stir in a dollop of plain Greek yogurt and mash the lamb and chickpeas.

FOR EVERYBODY ELSE Season with a pinch of salt and ground black pepper. Stir in the almonds, then sprinkle over the lemon rind and chopped fresh coriander. Serve with couscous or brown basmati rice and orange, red onion and black olive salad.

ORANGE, RED ONION & BLACK OLIVE SALAD
Zest one of the oranges and place the grated rind in a bowl. Peel both oranges and slice the flesh crossways into rounds.

Add the oil, lemon juice and vinegar to the grated rind, season with a pinch of salt and ground black pepper and whisk to make a dressing.

Arrange the orange slices on a platter, scatter over the red onion and olives and drizzle over the dressing.

AUBERGINE WITH LAMB

If you're stuck for something different then try this stuffed aubergine dish, which has aromatic Middle Eastern flavours that both your baby and your family will love. Adding the extra pine nuts and pomegranate seeds to everybody but the baby's portion really brings it to life.

Preparation time: 15 mins
Cooking time: 20 mins
Serves 2 and your baby

INGREDIENTS

2 large aubergines, halved lengthways

1 tbsp (15ml) olive oil

1 onion, peeled and finely chopped

½ tsp (2.5ml) ground cumin

½ tsp (2.5ml) paprika

½ tsp (2.5ml) ground cinnamon

200g lean minced lamb

1 tbsp (15ml) tomato purée

ADDITIONAL INGREDIENTS

2 tbsp pine nuts

2 tbsp (30ml) pomegranate seeds

A handful of flat leaf parsley, chopped

Rocket, to serve

Preheat the oven to 220ºC (Gas 7). Place the aubergine in a roasting tray skin side down, lightly smear with some of the olive oil and roast for 20 minutes.

Meanwhile, heat the remaining oil in a pan, add the onion, lamb and spices and cook over a medium heat for about 10 minutes, until the onions are softened. Add the tomato purée and cook for a further 6–8 minutes.

Remove the aubergines from the oven and cut one half in half for your baby.

FOR BABY Finely dice the aubergine, place it in a bowl with 2 tbsp (30ml) of the lamb mixture and stir together.

FOR EVERYBODY ELSE Divide the remaining lamb mixture between the aubergine halves, then scatter over the pine nuts, pomegranate seeds and the parsley. Serve on a bed of rocket.

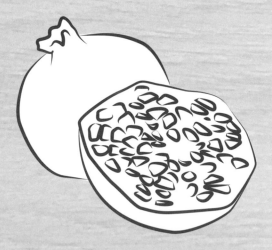

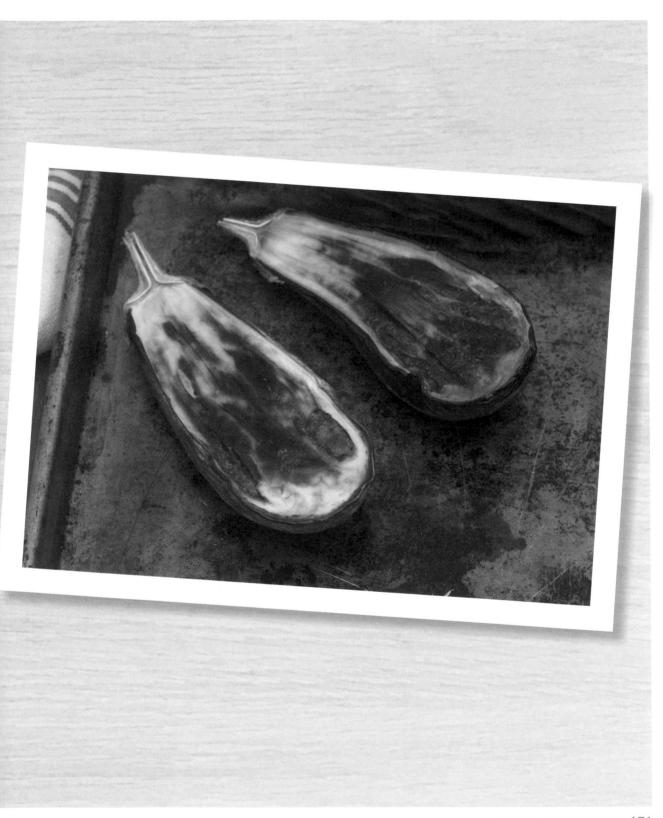

MOUSSAKA

Preparation time: 25 mins
Cooking time: 35-40 mins
Serves 4 and your baby

INGREDIENTS

2 tbsp (30ml) olive oil

1 onion, peeled and chopped

3 garlic cloves, peeled and chopped

500g lamb mince

150ml grape juice

1 tbsp (15ml) tomato purée

2 x 400g cans chopped tomatoes

1 tsp (5ml) dried oregano

1 tsp (5ml) ground allspice

1 cinnamon stick, snapped in half

A pinch of cumin seeds

3 aubergines, sliced

A pinch of salt and ground black pepper

75g butter

75g plain flour

600ml milk

1 egg yolk

3 tbsp (45ml) Parmesan cheese, grated

A pinch of nutmeg

Chunky parsley and mint salad,
to serve (for everybody apart from baby)

CHUNKY PARSLEY & MINT SALAD

½ cucumber, diced

1 beef tomato, diced

A handful of parsley leaves, torn

A handful of mint leaves, torn

Juice of ½ lemon

1 tsp (5ml) sesame seeds

You'll need a bit of time to make this, but it's worth the effort and you could easily make double the quantity and freeze half. The soft aubergines and white sauce give a lovely smooth texture for your baby and there are plenty of rich flavours for her to try. For everybody else, serve this sharp parsley and mint salad alongside, which will contrast perfectly with the creaminess of the moussaka.

Heat half the oil in a large pan, add the onion and garlic and cook gently for about 10 minutes, until the onion has softened. Add the lamb mince to the pan and cook until the meat is soft and cooked through.

Add the grape juice, tomato purée, chopped tomatoes, oregano, allspice, cinnamon stick and cumin seeds. Simmer, uncovered, over a very low heat for 1½ hours, stirring occasionally. Remove the cinnamon stick.

Heat the remaining oil in a frying pan over a medium heat and fry the aubergine slices until golden on both sides. Remove from the pan and drain on kitchen paper. Season with ground black pepper.

Preheat the oven to 190°C (Gas 5). To make the white sauce, melt the butter in a pan. Add the flour and cook for 30 seconds, stirring until the mixture forms a smooth paste. Gradually stir in the milk, beating constantly to avoid lumps, then bring to the boil, still stirring or whisking continuously and simmer for about 5 minutes, until thick. Remove from the heat and stir in the egg yolk, grated Parmesan and nutmeg.

To assemble the moussaka, place a layer of aubergine in the bottom of an ovenproof dish, followed by half the mince mixture. Add another layer of aubergine, the rest of the mince and a final layer of aubergine. Top with the white sauce and bake in the oven for 25–30 minutes.

FOR BABY Remove your baby's portion and gently mash with a fork.

FOR EVERYBODY ELSE Serve the moussaka with the chunky parsley and mint salad.

CHUNKY PARSLEY AND MINT SALAD

Place the cucumber, tomato and herbs in a bowl, squeeze over the lemon juice, toss together and sprinkle on the sesame seeds.

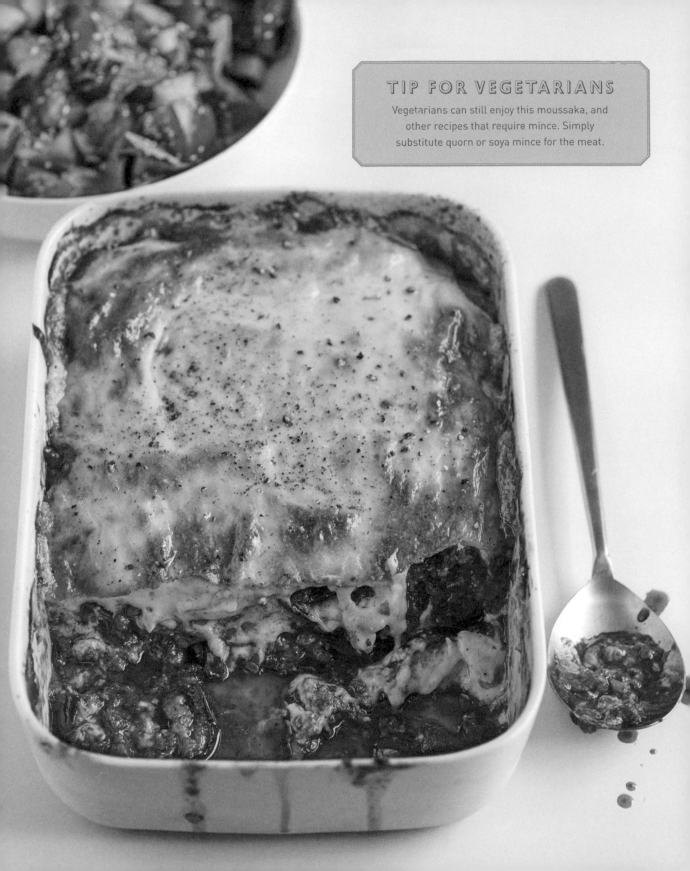

TIP FOR VEGETARIANS

Vegetarians can still enjoy this moussaka, and other recipes that require mince. Simply substitute quorn or soya mince for the meat.

BEEF AND JERUSALEM ARTICHOKE STEW

This is a great dish to make in the morning if you have a busy day ahead and know you'll resort to ready-made baby food for your baby and a takeaway for you if there isn't anything tasty waiting for you when you come home. Four hours of cooking means the meat will be melt in the mouth tender and easy to mash.

Preparation time: 15 mins
Cooking time: 3-4 hours
Serves 4 and your baby

INGREDIENTS
2 tbsp (30ml) olive oil

900g lean beef steak, diced

Flour, for dusting

6 shallots, peeled and quartered

2 large carrots, peeled and diced

4 Jerusalem artichokes, peeled and diced

2 parsnips, peeled and diced

½ butternut squash, peeled and diced

1 large sweet potato, peeled and diced

A handful of fresh sage

500ml alcohol-free red wine or grape juice

300ml beef stock

2 tbsp (30ml) tomato purée

Preheat the oven to 150°C (Gas 2). Heat the oil in a large casserole. Toss the meat in the flour and add it to the casserole with all the other ingredients.

Cover with a lid and cook in the oven for 3–4 hours.

FOR BABY Remove your baby's portion and gently mash with a fork.

FOR EVERYBODY ELSE Just serve it as it is!

MUSHROOMS, IN A STEW!

Often with stews there is too much left over to simply discard but not enough to provide another meal. A great way to bulk out meaty stews without having to add more meat is to use mushrooms instead. They work brilliantly to give the same texture and add a subtle flavour. Chop 4-5 large mushrooms into meat sized chunks, sauté them in a little olive oil and a pat of butter and then stir into the leftover stew and reheat everything together. You can also finely chopped mushrooms to go with mince to make a bolognaise sauce or chilli con carne, or they work well along with diced chicken for stir frys or casseroles.

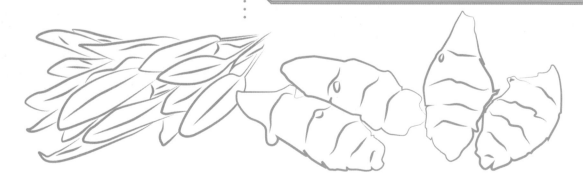

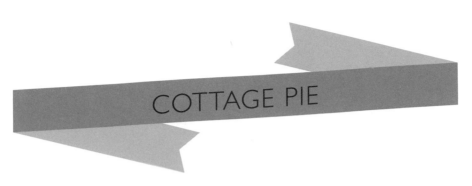

COTTAGE PIE

Another loved family classic with a little twist, this dish combines celeriac with potato to make the creamy mash topping. The celeriac adds more fibre and helps lower the GI. Worcestershire sauce is usually added when cooking the mince, but as it is salty it's best not to use it for your baby. Instead, add it to the side of leeks for a flavour kick.

Preparation time: 20 mins
Cooking time: 50-60 mins
Serves 4 and your baby

INGREDIENTS
2 tbsp (30ml) olive oil

500g minced beef

1 large onion, peeled and diced

2 celery sticks, finely chopped

2 carrots, peeled and diced

400g canned chopped tomatoes

2 tbsp (30ml) tomato purée

1 bay leaf

1 tsp (5ml) chopped fresh thyme leaves

300ml low-salt vegetable stock

500g celeriac, peeled and diced

500g potato, peeled and diced

1 tbsp (15ml) butter

100g crème fraîche

Ground black pepper

ADDITIONAL INGREDIENTS
A pat of butter

1 leek, thinly sliced

1 tbsp (15ml) Worcestershire sauce

1 tbsp (15ml) Parmesan cheese

Preheat the oven to 200°C (Gas 6). Heat the oil in a large pan, add the beef mince and brown all over. Add the onion, celery and carrots and cook for about 10 minutes, until softened.

Stir in the chopped tomatoes, tomato purée, bay leaf, thyme leaves and stock. Cover and simmer for 30 minutes, stirring occasionally.

To make the topping, bring a large pan of water to the boil and cook the celeriac and potato for 8–10 minutes, until soft. Drain well and tip into a large bowl. Add the butter and crème fraîche and mash until smooth, then season with a little black pepper.

Pour the cooked mince mixture into a shallow ovenproof dish and top with mash. Bake in the oven for 20–30 minutes, until the top is golden brown.

FOR BABY Remove their portion and serve.

FOR EVERYBODY ELSE Just before the cottage pie is ready, heat the butter in a pan and gently sauté the leeks over a medium heat. Add the Worcestershire sauce and Parmesan and serve on the side with the pie.

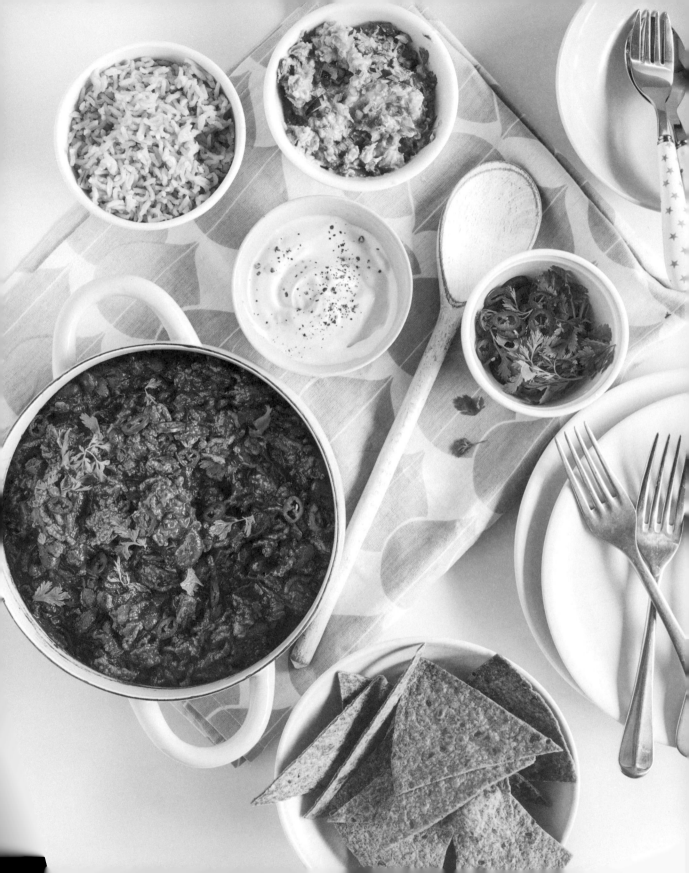

CHILLI CON CARNE

Preparation time: 30 mins
Cooking time: 2–3 hours
Serves 4 and your baby

INGREDIENTS

2 tbsp (30ml) rapeseed oil

500g beef mince

1 red onion, peeled and finely chopped

1 celery stick, chopped

½ tsp (2.5ml) chilli powder

1 tsp (5ml) dried oregano

400g canned chopped tomatoes

300ml low-salt beef stock

400g canned kidney beans, rinsed and drained

ADDITIONAL INGREDIENTS

Salt and ground black pepper

50g plain chocolate (minimum 70 per cent cocoa solids), roughly chopped

1 red chilli, deseeded and finely sliced

A handful of fresh coriander leaves, chopped

To serve

Cooked brown basmati rice

Sour cream or crème fraîche

Seeded wholegrain tortilla chips and quick guacamole (for everybody apart from baby)

QUICK GUACAMOLE

2 ripe avocados

1 green chilli, deseeded and finely chopped

½ red onion, peeled and finely chopped

1 tsp (5ml) ground cumin

A handful of fresh coriander, finely chopped

Juice of 1 lime

A pinch of salt

Here's a lovely family feast for a Saturday night: a delicious slow-cooked soft chilli with mashed beans and cool yogurt for your baby and lots of picky bits for everyone else. After you have removed your baby's portion, spice up the meat with fresh chilli to your taste and then melt in the dark chocolate to add extra richness.

Preheat the oven to 150°C (Gas 2). Heat half the oil over a medium-high heat in a large flameproof casserole. Add the beef mince and fry until browned all over. Remove from the pan with a slotted spoon and set aside.

Add the remaining oil to the pan along with the onion and celery and fry for about 10 minutes, until softened. Stir in the chilli powder and oregano until well combined. Cook for a further 2 minutes.

Return the mince to the pan, then stir in the tomatoes, stock and kidney beans. Bring to the boil, then reduce the heat and cover with a tight-fitting lid. Place in the preheated oven and cook for 2–3 hours.

FOR BABY Remove your baby's portion, mash the beans gently with a fork and stir in a dollop of sour cream or crème fraîche and 2 tbsp (30ml) of the cooked brown basmati rice.

FOR EVERYBODY ELSE Remove from the oven, then taste and adjust the seasoning. Stir in the chocolate pieces until they have just melted, then scatter over the chopped chilli and fresh coriander. Serve with all the accompaniments.

QUICK GUACAMOLE

Halve the avocados, remove the stones and slice the flesh. Reserve some of the slices to give to your baby to hold. Place the rest in a bowl, mash with a fork, add the rest of the ingredients and mix well together.

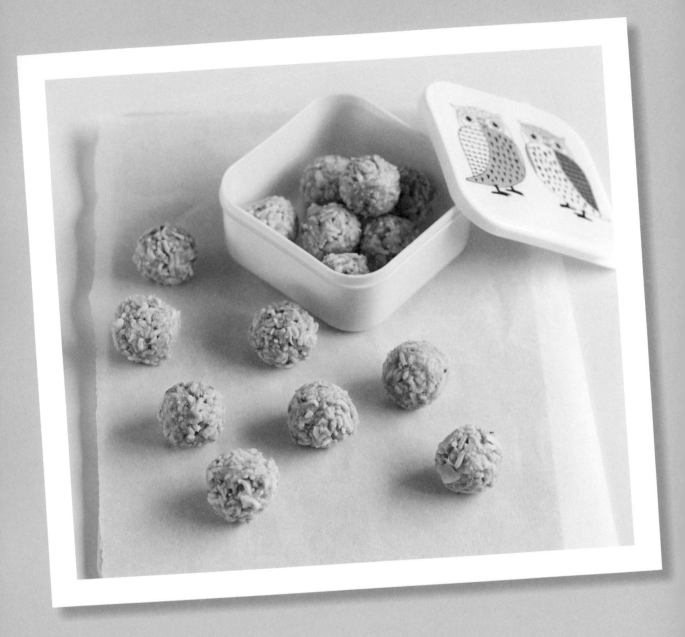
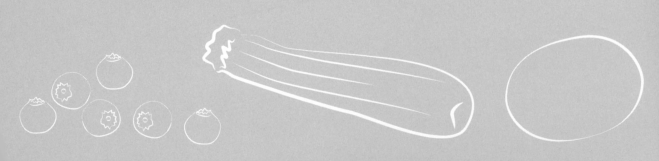

NATURALLY SWEET TREATS

These refined-sugar-free treats are hugely worth the effort.
Identify a little window of time, maybe while your baby is taking a nap,
and make a batch of a few of the recipes you fancy. Many of them keep
well in an airtight container or can be frozen, meaning it's easy to grab
a couple of these snacks from the freezer, toss them into your change
bag and they will be defrosted by the time you're ready to enjoy them.
As your baby gets older and can manage finger foods you can
share these delicious snacks and help prevent your baby from
developing a sweet tooth by avoiding giving them processed
foods or recipes packed with refined sugars.

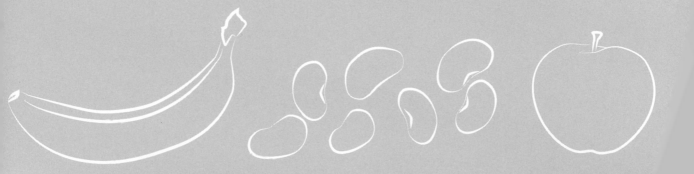

CHEESE AND APPLE SCONES

Cheese and apple is one of my favourite combinations and it works fantastically in these deliciously light scones. They are just the thing to go with your cup of tea at the end of a busy day.

Preparation time: 15 mins
Cooking time: 30 mins
Makes 12

INGREDIENTS

180g self-raising wholemeal flour

125g butter, diced, plus extra for spreading (optional)

150g Cheddar cheese, grated

2 apples, peeled, cored and finely diced

3 eggs, beaten

Preheat the oven to 180°C (Gas 4). Grease a 12-hole muffin tin.

Sift the flour into a mixing bowl, adding the bran pieces left in the sieve to the bowl. Add the diced butter and rub into the flour with your fingertips until the mixture looks like coarse crumbs. Gently stir in most of the cheese (leave a little to sprinkle on top) and the diced apple.

Add the beaten eggs to the flour mixture and stir with a wooden spoon to make a stiff mixture.

Spoon the mixture evenly into each muffin hole. Sprinkle with the reserved grated cheese and bake for 30 minutes, until golden and cooked through.

Remove from the oven and leave to cool in the tin for about 10 minutes, then turn them out on to a cooling rack. Serve warm or cold, perhaps spread with a little butter.

Store leftovers in an airtight container for up to 2–3 days, or open-freeze them on a baking sheet before transferring to a freezer bag. To thaw, remove however many scones you require from the freezer and let them defrost at room temperature. For best results, however, put the still-frozen scones on a baking sheet and thaw and reinvigorate them in a low oven set to 160°C (Gas 3) for about 15 minutes.

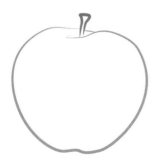

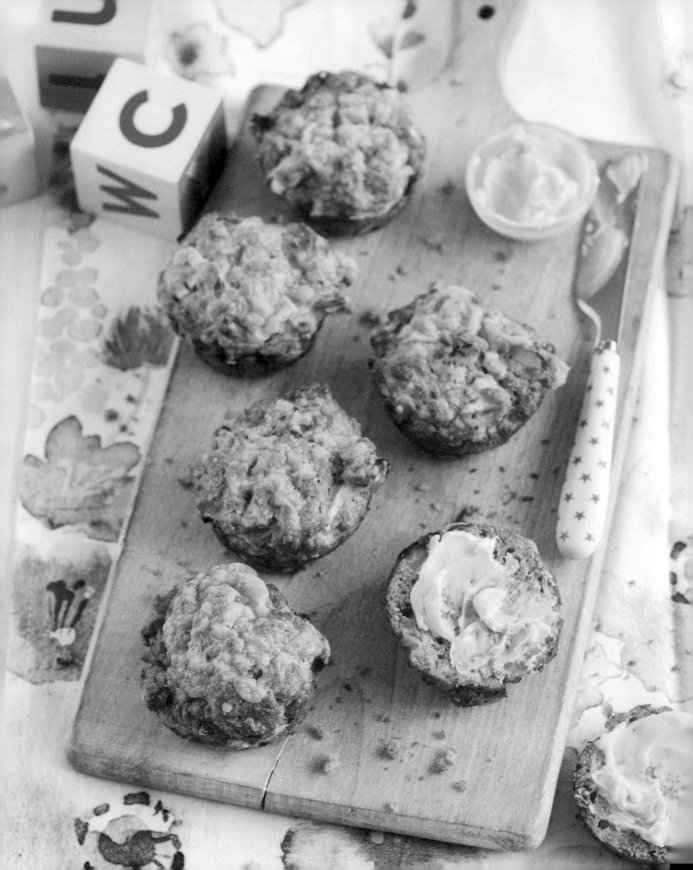

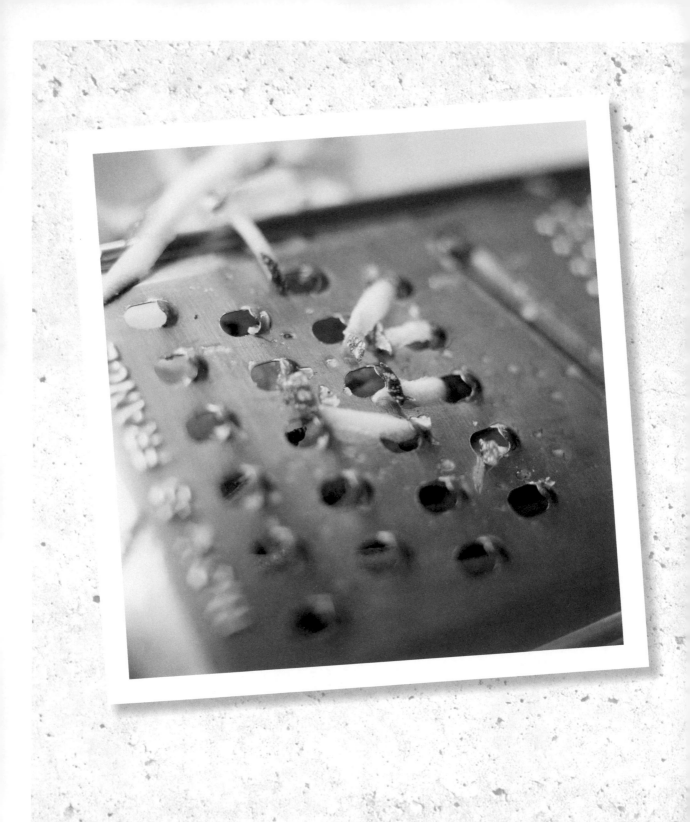

COURGETTE MUFFINS

These are light and moist, the courgette adds bulk without calories and the apple and orange juice gives them a subtle flavour, while the pumpkin seeds add a satisfying crunch.

Preparation time: 15 mins
Cooking time: 12-15 mins
Makes 12

INGREDIENTS
50g pumpkin seeds
3 tbsp (45ml) butter
1 courgette
1 apple
Juice from 1 orange
1 egg
300g spelt flour
1 tsp (5ml) baking powder
1 tsp (5ml) mixed spice

Preheat the oven to 220ºC (Gas 7). Line a muffin tray with paper cases.

Place the pumpkin seeds in a plastic food bag and crush with a rolling pin.

Melt the butter in a small pan or in the microwave, then leave to cool slightly. Grate the courgette and apple into a bowl and stir in the orange juice. Beat the egg, then stir it into the grated courgette and apple. Add the melted butter and stir well.

Sift the flour and baking powder into a separate bowl, add the mixed spice and gradually stir the wet mixture into the dry mixture until sticky and well combined. Stir in the pumpkin seeds.

Divide the mixture among the muffin cases in the muffin tray. Bake for 12-15 minutes, or until a skewer inserted into the centre of the muffins comes out clean.

Remove from the oven and leave to cool in the tin for about 10 minutes, then turn out on to a cooling rack. Serve warm or cold.

Store leftovers in an airtight container for up to 2-3 days, or open-freeze them on a baking sheet before transferring to a freezer bag. To thaw, remove however many muffins you require from the freezer and let them defrost at room temperature. For best results, however, put the still-frozen muffins on a baking sheet and thaw and reinvigorate them in a low oven at 160ºC (Gas 3) for about 15 minutes.

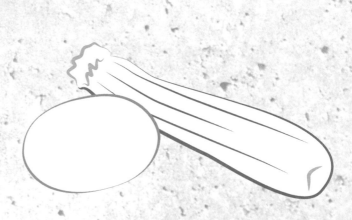

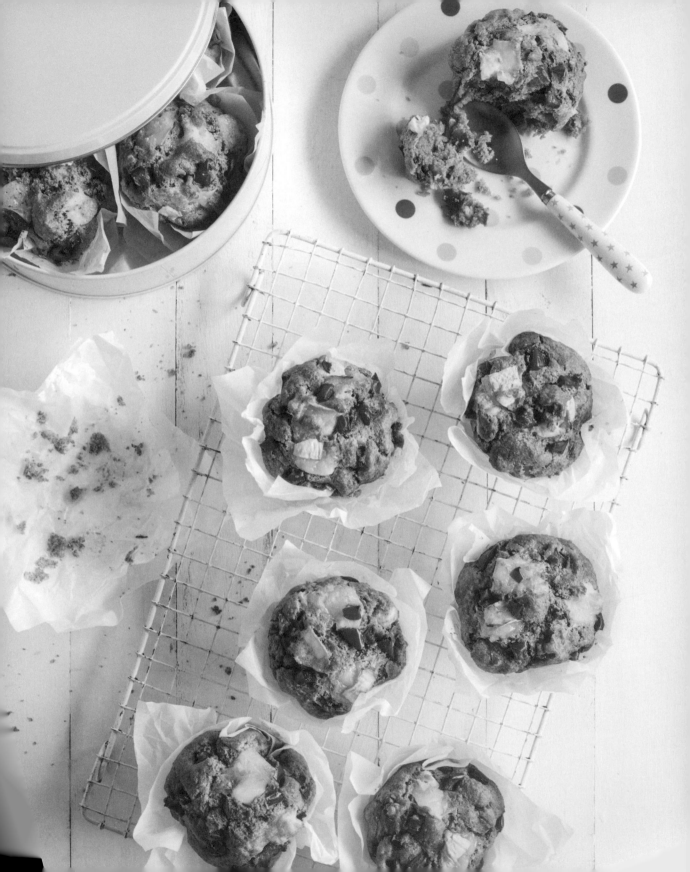

PEPPER AND GOAT'S CHEESE MUFFINS

If you're craving something salty, before you open a big bag of crisps try one of these muffins. They have a sharp savoury flavour that will satisfy the craving. If you like them more spicy, simply double the amount of cayenne pepper.

Preparation time: 15 mins
Cooking time: 30 mins
Makes 12

INGREDIENTS

300g wholemeal flour

2 tsp (10ml) baking powder

1 tsp (5ml) bicarbonate of soda

½ tsp (2.5ml) cayenne pepper

1 red pepper, deseeded and diced

150g goat's cheese, diced

1 egg, beaten

225ml milk

100ml sunflower oil

Preheat the oven to 190°C (Gas 5). Grease a 12-hole muffin tin.

Sift the flour, baking powder and bicarbonate of soda into a bowl, adding the bran pieces left in the sieve to the bowl and stir in the cayenne pepper.

Add the diced pepper and cheese and mix thoroughly using a wooden spoon. Make a well in the centre.

Mix together the beaten egg, milk and oil in a jug and pour gradually into the flour mixture, stirring with a wooden spoon, until combined.

Spoon the mixture evenly into the muffin tin. Bake in the oven for 30 minutes, until golden brown and a skewer inserted into the centre of the muffins comes out clean.

Remove from the oven and leave to cool in the tin for about 10 minutes, then turn out on to a cooling rack. Serve warm or cold.

Store leftovers in an airtight container for up to 2–3 days, or open-freeze them on a baking sheet before transferring to a freezer bag. To thaw, remove however many muffins you require from the freezer and let them defrost at room temperature. For best results, however, put the still-frozen scones on a baking sheet and thaw and reinvigorate them in a low oven at 160°C (Gas 3) for about 15 minutes.

BLUEBERRY PANCAKES

These are perfect for a weekend brunch. The banana gives them a natural sweetness and the oats make them satisfying and filling, so you won't be looking to snack later on.

Preparation time: 10 mins
Cooking time: 10-15 mins
Makes about 8

INGREDIENTS
90g rolled oats

1 tsp (5ml) baking powder

150ml plain Greek yogurt

1 banana

2 eggs

2–3 drops vanilla extract

A splash of milk or almond milk (optional)

Butter, for greasing

A small punnet (about 150g) of blueberries

Place the oats, baking powder, yogurt, banana, eggs and vanilla extract into a blender and blend until smooth. You may need to add a splash of milk or almond milk if the batter is too thick. Set the batter aside to thicken up for a few minutes. It should have the consistency of double cream.

Using a piece of kitchen paper and a dab of butter, lightly coat a large non-stick skillet or griddle with fat and heat over a medium-low heat. Drop 2 tbsp (30ml) of batter on to the skillet or griddle and put a few blueberries on top of each. Cook until bubbles appear on top of the pancake.

Flip over the pancakes and cook until golden brown on the underside. Transfer to a plate and cover with a clean tea towel to keep warm.

Wipe the skillet or griddle clean with kitchen paper, re-grease and repeat with the remaining batter.

Enjoy the pancakes immediately. You can keep leftovers on a plate, covered with cling film, in the refrigerator overnight, then simply reheat the pancakes in the microwave for about 30 seconds, or in a low oven for a few minutes.

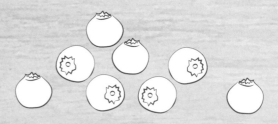

BANANA AND OATMEAL PANCAKES

Use mixed spice instead of the vanilla for a stronger flavoured pancake and make them more substantial by adding the cheese with the fruit.

Preparation time:10 mins
Cooking time: 10-15 mins
Makes about 8

INGREDIENTS
90g rolled oats

1 banana

2–3 drops vanilla extract

1 tsp (5ml) baking powder

1 tsp (5ml) mixed spice

1 large egg

4 tbsp (60ml) milk

Butter, for greasing

100g soft cheese

100g raspberries

Place all of the ingredients, except the butter, cheese and raspberries, in a blender and blend for about 30 seconds, until completely smooth.

Using a piece of kitchen paper and a dab of butter, lightly coat a large non-stick skillet or griddle with fat and heat over a medium-low heat. Drop 2 tbsp (30ml) of batter on to the skillet or griddle.

Place the soft cheese into a bowl and fold in the fruit. You may need to give the cheese a whisk with a fork to loosen it before you can gently stir in the raspberries; try to avoid crushing them.

Cook the pancakes until bubbles appear on top. Flip them over and cook until golden brown on the underside. Transfer to a plate and cover with a clean tea towel to keep warm.

Wipe the skillet or griddle clean with kitchen paper, re-grease and repeat with the remaining batter.

Serve immediately with dollops of the cheese and fruit mixture.

You can keep leftovers on a plate, covered with cling film, in the refrigerator overnight, then simply reheat the pancakes in the microwave for about 30 seconds, or in a low oven for a few minutes.

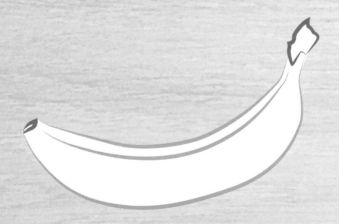

QUINOA AND BLUEBERRY PANCAKES

Try the same recipe with quinoa flour instead of the oats. Quinoa has a slightly nuttier flavour and is higher in protein to help you feel fuller for longer.

Preparation time: 10 mins
Cooking time: 10-15 mins
Makes about 8

INGREDIENTS
140g quinoa flour

1 tsp (5ml) baking powder

½ tsp (2.5ml) bicarbonate of soda

1 large ripe banana, mashed

150ml plain Greek yogurt

1 egg, slightly beaten

2–3 drops vanilla extract

4 tbsp (60ml) milk, plus more if necessary

200g blueberries

Butter, for greasing

Mix together the quinoa flour, baking powder and bicarbonate of soda in a large bowl.

In a separate bowl, use an electric whisk to beat together the banana, yogurt, egg, vanilla extract and milk, until smooth and well combined.

Add the wet ingredients to the flour mixture and mix together. If the batter is too thick, loosen it with a splash of extra milk. It should have the consistency of double cream. Fold in the blueberries.

Using a piece of kitchen paper and a dab of butter, lightly coat a large non-stick skillet or griddle with fat and heat over a medium-low heat. Drop 2 tbsp (30ml) of batter on to the skillet or griddle. Spread out with the back of a spoon. Cook until bubbles appear on top and the edges are well cooked.

Flip over the pancakes and cook for about 2 minutes, until golden brown on the underside. Transfer to a plate and cover with a clean tea towel to keep warm.

Wipe the skillet or griddle clean with kitchen paper, re-grease and repeat with the remaining batter.

Enjoy the pancakes immediately. You can keep leftovers on a plate, covered with cling film, in the refrigerator overnight, then simply reheat the pancakes in the microwave for about 30 seconds, or in a low oven for a few minutes.

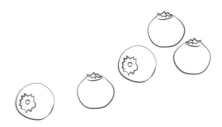

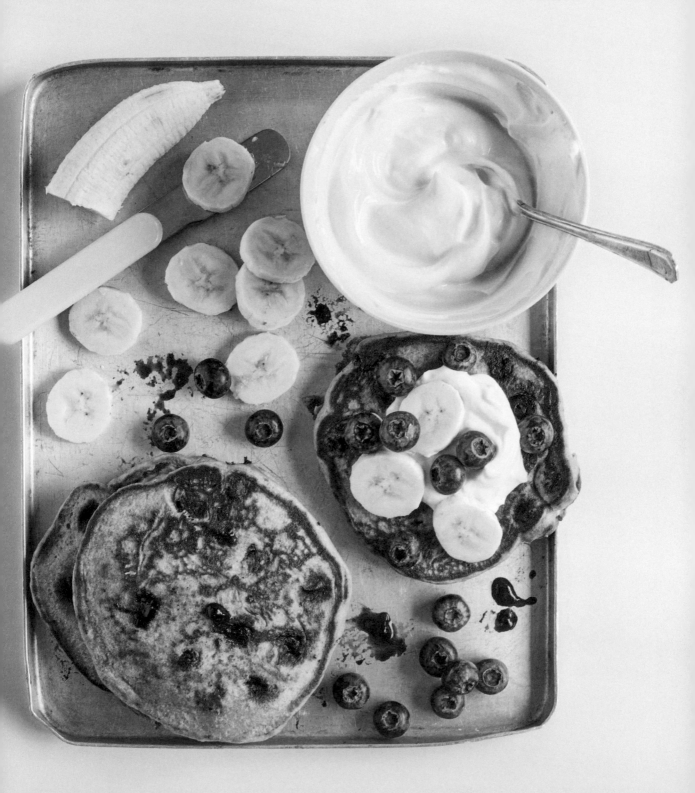

CARROT AND CINNAMON CUPCAKES

These cupcakes have a wonderful texture and colour thanks to the carrot and as you lose your sweet tooth, you'll find the raisins and orange zest make them just sweet enough.

Preparation time: 15 mins
Cooking time: 15 mins
Makes 12

INGREDIENTS

150g spelt flour

100g ground almonds

75g raisins

2 tsp (10ml) cinnamon

1 tsp (5ml) ground mixed spice

1 tsp (5ml) baking powder

1 tsp (5ml) bicarbonate of soda

3 large eggs

100ml sunflower oil

3 tbsp (45ml) milk

300g carrots, coarsely grated

150g soft cheese

Grated rind of 1 orange

Preheat the oven to 180ºC (Gas 4). Line a 12-hole muffin tin with paper cases.

Put the flour, almonds, raisins, cinnamon, mixed spice, baking powder and bicarbonate of soda in a large bowl and mix thoroughly. Make a well in the centre.

In a separate bowl, whisk the eggs, oil and milk together and stir in the grated carrot. Add the egg mixture to the dry ingredients, stirring to form a thick batter.

Spoon the mixture into the paper cases until they are two-thirds full. Bake for 10–15 minutes, or until golden-brown on top and a skewer inserted into one of the cakes comes out clean.

Remove from the oven and set aside to cool for 10 minutes, then remove the cakes from the tin and cool completely on a wire rack.

Stir the cheese and orange zest together and spread evenly over the cakes.

Store leftovers in an airtight container in the fridge for up to 2–3 days. You can also open-freeze the un-iced cakes on a baking sheet, then transfer them to a freezer bag. To thaw, remove however many cakes you require from the freezer and let them defrost at room temperature before icing.

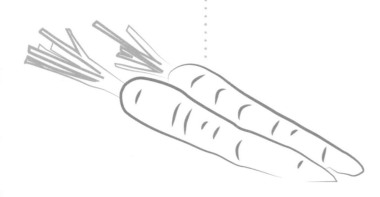

APPLE AND BLACKBERRY LOAF

This is a delicious loaf kept moist by the apple and packed
full of flavour from the blackberries.

Preparation time: 15 mins
Cooking time: 75-80 mins
Makes 1 loaf

INGREDIENTS

175g butter, plus extra for greasing

250g wholemeal spelt flour,
plus 1 tbsp (15ml) for dusting

1 tsp (5ml) ground mixed spice

1 tsp (5ml) baking powder

1 tsp (5ml) bicarbonate of soda

2 eggs

2 apples, peeled and grated

200g blackberries

Preheat the oven to 180ºC (Gas 4). Butter a loaf tin and line the bottom.

In a large bowl, rub the butter and flour together with your fingertips to make fine crumbs. Gently stir in the mixed spice, baking powder and bicarbonate of soda.

Whisk the eggs in a bowl and stir in the grated apple. Add the wet mixture to the flour mixture and lightly stir in, being careful not to over-mix.

Dust the blackberries in the 1 tbsp (15ml) flour and shake to ensure they are coated. This helps to prevent the berries from sinking to the bottom of the cake. Gently fold in the berries to the mixture with a metal spoon.

Spoon the cake mixture into the tin and level off. Bake for 1 hour 15 minutes–1 hour 20 minutes, or until a skewer inserted into the centre comes out clean. Start checking the cake after 50 minutes and cover the top loosely with foil if it is browning too much.

Remove from the oven and set aside to cool in the tin for 10 minutes, then remove the cake from the tin and cool completely on a wire rack.

Store leftovers in an airtight container for up to 2–3 days, or cut the remaining cake into slices and open-freeze them on a baking sheet before transferring to a freezer bag. To thaw, remove however many slices you require from the freezer and let them defrost at room temperature.

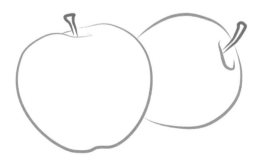

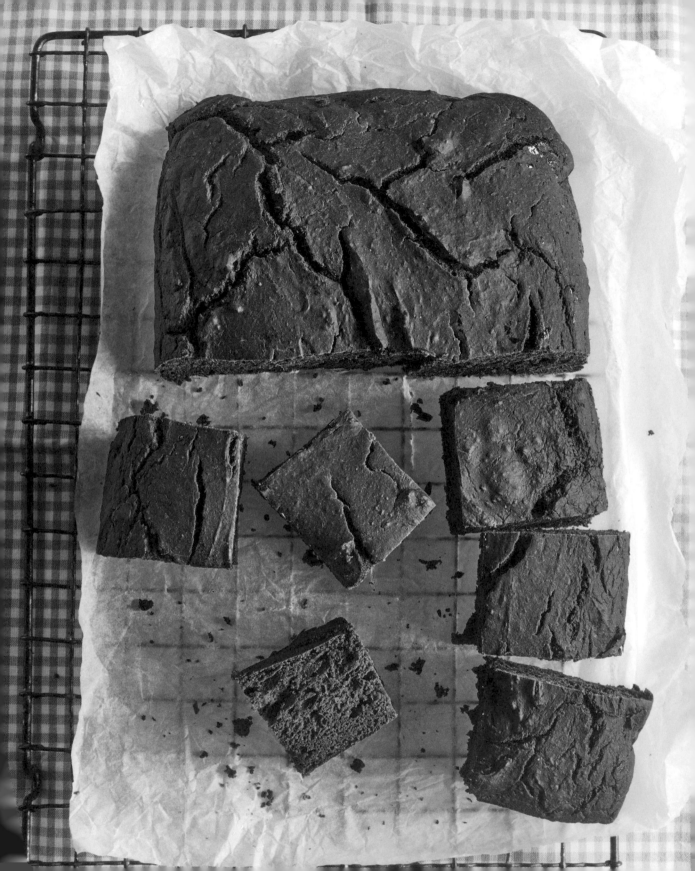

BUTTER BEAN BROWNIES

Butter beans may not be the first thing you think of for a brownie, but the addition of the beans provides a lovely moist texture and boosts the fibre content making them filling and satisfying.

Preparation time: 20 mins
Cooking time: 40-45 mins
Makes 16

INGREDIENTS

Butter or oil, for greasing

400g canned butter beans, rinsed and drained

1–2 tbsp (15–30ml) water

250g apple sauce

200g self-raising flour

2 tsp (10ml) baking powder

3 tbsp (45ml) cocoa powder

3 eggs

A few drops of vanilla extract

6 dates, finely chopped

Preheat the oven to 180°C (Gas 4) and lightly grease a 26 x 18cm baking or traybake tin.

Place the beans and water in a food processor and whizz together until smooth – you are looking for the consistency of mashed potato. Add more water if the mixture looks too dry. Add the apple sauce and process again for 1–2 minutes, until smooth and well combined.

Sift the flour, baking powder and cocoa powder into a large bowl. In a separate bowl, beat the eggs. Add one-third of the bean mixture to the egg mixture together with one-third of the flour mixture and fold in carefully. Repeat twice more until all the ingredients are gently incorporated.

Add the vanilla extract and dates and gently fold through. Pour the mixture into the baking or traybake tin and spread evenly.

Bake for 40–45 minutes, until a skewer inserted in the middle comes out clean. Remove from the oven and set aside to cool for 10 minutes, then turn out on to a wire rack to cool completely before cutting the brownie into squares.

Store leftovers in an airtight container for up to 2–3 days, or open-freeze the squares on a baking sheet before transferring to a freezer bag. To thaw, remove however many squares you require from the freezer and let them defrost at room temperature.

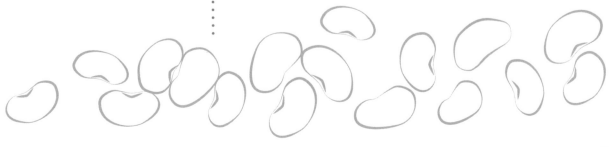

APRICOT OATCAKES

These lovely oatcakes are good enough to eat on their own,
but also delicious topped with a slice of cheese.

Preparation time: 10 mins
Cooking time: 20-30 mins
Makes about 15

INGREDIENTS

225g rolled oats, plus extra for rolling out

60g spelt flour, plus extra for rolling out

½ tsp (2.5ml) bicarbonate of soda

60g butter

100g dried apricot pieces

4-5 tbsp (60-75ml) hot water

Preheat the oven to 190ºC (Gas 5).

In a large bowl, mix together the oats, flour and bicarbonate of soda. Add the butter and rub together until everything is mixed and has the consistency of large breadcrumbs. Add the dried apricot pieces.

Add the water little by litte and combine until you have a thick dough. The amount of water required varies depending on the oats.

Sprinkle some extra flour and oats on a work surface and roll out the dough to a thickness of about 5mm. Use a cookie cutter to cut out shapes.

Place the oatcakes on a baking tray and bake for 20–30 minutes, or until slightly golden brown.

Store leftovers in an airtight container for up to 2–3 days.

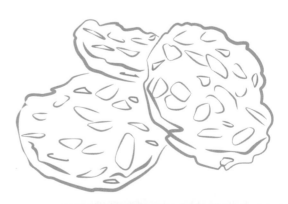

GRANOLA BITES

This clever recipe uses egg white instead of sugar as the glue for the grains and nuts.
Stir into Greek yogurt and add a handful of berries.

Preparation time: 10 mins
Cooking time: 50 m ins
Makes about 350g

INGREDIENTS

250g rolled oats

100g ground almonds

1 tbsp (15ml) toasted wheat germ

2 tbsp (30ml) olive or rapeseed oil

1 tsp (5ml) cinnamon

1 large egg white

Preheat the oven to 150°C (Gas 2).

Combine all the ingredients except the egg white in a large bowl, tossing to coat evenly.

Whisk the egg white in a small bowl until frothy, then stir into the granola mixture, distributing it throughout.

Spread the mixture in a single layer on a parchment-lined baking sheet.

Bake the mixture for 50 minutes. About halfway through the baking time, use a large spatula to carefully turn over sections of the granola, retaining large clumps.

When it is evenly browned and feels dry to the touch, remove from the oven and transfer to a cooling rack. Cool completely before breaking up into clusters.

Store in an airtight container for up to a month.

FRUITY FLAPJACKS

These are great for out and about snacks, packed full of energy
so you won't need that bar of chocolate.

Preparation time: 20 mins
Cooking time: 25 mins
Makes 20

INGREDIENTS
**5 tbsp (75ml) vegetable oil,
plus extra for greasing**

2 bananas, peeled

175g ready-to-eat dates, chopped

180g porridge oats

1 tsp (5ml) vanilla extract

Preheat the oven to 190ºC (Gas 5). Grease a 20 x 20cm baking tin.
    Mash the bananas in a large bowl. Add the dates and oil to the banana and mix together.
    Stir in the oats and the vanilla extract and leave for 5 minutes, so the oats absorb the oil.
    Spoon the mixture into the tin and press down the surface with the back of a spatula so it binds well. Bake for 25 minutes, until set and golden brown.
    Remove from the oven and allow to cool in the tin until just warm, then turn it out and cut it into squares. Doing this while the flapjack is still slightly warm makes turning it out much easier and helps to prevent it from shattering when you cut it.
    Store leftovers in an airtight container for up to 4–5 days.

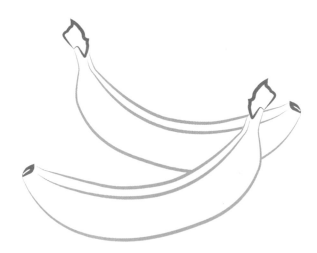

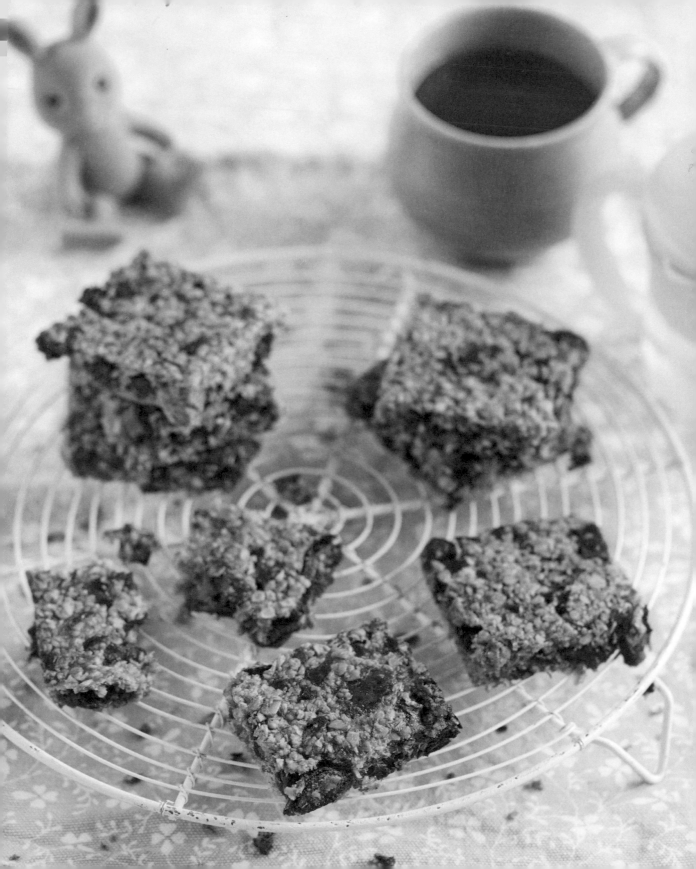

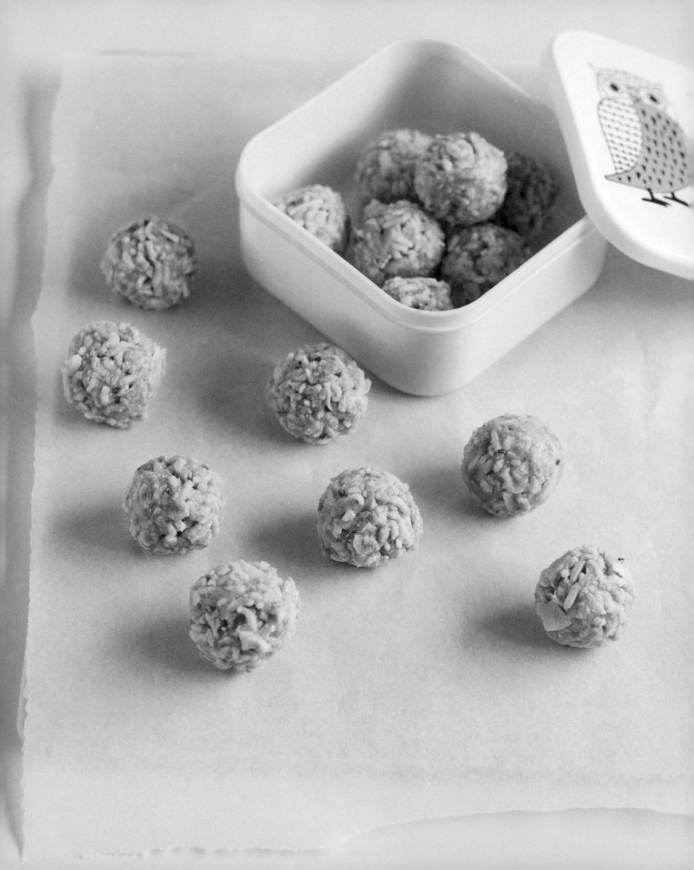

NUT BUTTER AND RICE BALLS

Another really good little snack when you need an energy boost. They are packed full of vitamins and slow release energy that will satisfy hunger pangs and keep you going on busy days.

Preparation time: 10 mins
Cooking time: 0 mins
Makes 12-16

INGREDIENTS

4 tbsp (60ml) peanut or other nut butter

1 tbsp (15ml) coconut oil

1 tsp (5ml) vanilla extract

1 tbsp (15ml) honey

2 tbsp (30ml) ground flaxseed

2 tbsp (30ml) small coconut flakes

250g cooked brown basmati rice and quinoa (a pouch is most convenient), cooled

In a large bowl, beat the peanut butter with the coconut oil to soften it, then stir in the vanilla extract and honey. Stir in the ground flaxseed, coconut flakes and cooled rice, until well combined. The mixture should be thick and sticky.

Freeze for about 10 minutes or until chilled. Use a spoon to scoop out even amounts and roll into balls about the size of a cherry tomato.

Store in the freezer, then simply remove a ball as required and leave it for about 10 minutes to thaw slightly before you eat it.

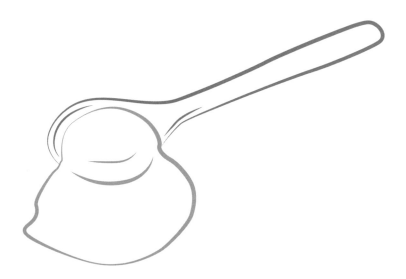

CONVERSION CHARTS

LIQUID/DRY MEASURES

U.S.	METRIC
¼ teaspoon	1.25 milliliters
½ teaspoon	2.5 milliliters
1 teaspoon	5 milliliters
1 tablespoon (3 teaspoons)	15 milliliters
1 fluid ounce (2 tablespoons)	30 milliliters
¼ cup	60 milliliters
⅓ cup	80 milliliters
½ cup	120 milliliters
1 cup	240 milliliters
1 pint	(2 cups) 480 milliliters
1 quart	(4 cups; 32 ounces) 960 milliliters
1 gallon	(4 quarts) 3.84 liters
1 ounce	(by weight) 28 grams
1 pound	454 grams
2.2 pounds	1 kilogram

OVEN TEMPERATURES

°F	GAS	MARK °C
250	½	120
275	1	40
300	2	150
325	3	165
350	4	180
375	5	190
400	6	200
425	7	220
450	8	230
475	9	240
500	10	260
550	Broil 2	90

Dedicated to Ronnie, Daniel and Jacob

ACKNOWLEDGEMENTS

I would like to thank the marvellous team at Bloomsbury for all their guidance and encouragement,especially Charlotte Croft and Sarah Skipper for their great input and advice. I would like to thank Tony Fitzpatrick for the many years of continued loyalty and support and always being at the end of the phone for those reassuring chats! Finally I would like to thank my wonderfully patient and supportive husband who gave me the confidence and time needed to write this book, and my two boys who were the inspiration behind it.

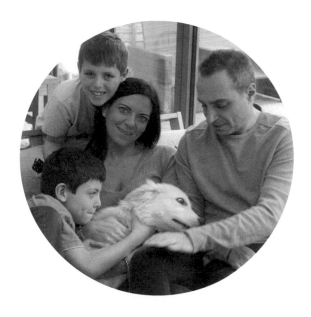

INDEX

Page numbers in *italics* are illustrations.